Traditional Chinese Medicine (TCM) is one of the great Chinese scientific heritages. Chinese patent formulas including simple and proved receipes are the successful cream of the long term clinical practices. This volume of Chinese patent medicines provides a collection of 355 efficiente valuable and most famous prescriptions among Chinese patent drugs. These patent medicines are organized in this book to six categories: medicine for internal disease. gynecopathy. pediatrics. surgical disease. the disease of five sense organs and health care. The introduction of these patent medicines includes their Chinese nomenclature and English translations. Also covered are their principle ingredients. functions. indications. directions and precautions. I hope that this specialized book would provide considerable to the Chinese patent medicine's usage in clinical practices. and contribute to the international academic communication between China and other countries. I am deeply indebted to Drs. Chen Kai. Zhang Qun-hao. Wang wei. Song Jun. Hsia I-szu. and Lin Yuxiong. Their editorial efforts did much to shape the scope of this book.

Chen Ke-ji. MD.
Professor of Medicine
Xiyuan Hospital. China Academy of Traditional Chinese Medicine.
Academician. Chinese Academy of Sciences

CONTENTS
目 录

I—2 Prescriptions for Heat-Clearing
清热剂

I—3 Prescriptions for Dispelling Wind
祛风剂）

I-5 **Prescriptions for Promoting Digestion**
（消导剂)

**I-15 Prescriptions for Inducing Astringency
固涩剂）**

**I-16 Prescriptions for Calming Endopathic Wind
熄风剂）**

III MEDICINE FOR PREDIATRICS

INDEX OF CHINESE ALPHABET

I Medicine for Internal Diseases
内 科 类

I-1 Prescriptions for Relieving External Syndrome
解表剂

001 YINQIAO JIEDU WAN (银翘解毒丸)

Antitoxic Bolus of Honeysuckle Flower and Forsythia

PRINCIPAL INGREDIENTS

Honeysuckle flower (Flos Lonicerae), Arctium fruit (Fructus Arctii), Forsythia fruit (Fructus Forsythiae), Platycodon root (Radix Platycodi), Peppermint (Herba Menthae), Lophantherum (Herba Lophatheri), Schizonepeta spike (Spica Schizonepetae), Liquorice (Radix Glycyrrhizae), Fermented soybean (Semen Sojiae Praeparata)

FUNCTIONS

Relieving the exterior syndrome with drugs pungent in flavor and cool in property, clearing away heat and toxic materials.

INDICATION

For the treatment of common cold, acute

· *1* ·

tonsillitis, encephalitis B, epidemic cerebrospinal meningitis and infection of upper respiratory of wind-heat type marked by fever, headache, cough, dry mouth and sore throat, red tip of the tongue with thin white or yellow fur, rapid pulse.

DIRECTIONS

To be taken orally, one pill each time, twice or three times a day.

PRECAUTION

Spicy and greasy food should be avoided to take.

002   SANGJU GANMAO PIAN (桑菊感冒片)

Tablet of Mulberry and Chrysanthemum for Common Cold

PRINCIPAL INGREDIENTS

Mulberry leaf (Folium Mori), Chrysanthemum flower (Flos Chrysanthemi), Bitter apricot kernel (Semen Armeniacae Amarum), Forsythia fruit (Fructus Forsythiae), Peppermint (Herba Menthae), Platycodon root (Radix Platycodi), Licorice root (Radix Glycyrrhizae), Reed rhizome (Rhizoma Phragmitis)

FUNCTIONS

Relieving the exterior syndrome with drugs

pungent in flavor and cool in property, facilitating the flow of the lung-Qi to relieve cough.

INDICATION

The onset of cough due to wind-heat, marked by cough, mild feverish body, slight thirst, thin and white coating of the tongue and floating pulse. It is also used to treat common cold, influenza, acute bronchitis, bronchial pneumonia and acute tonsillitis that indicate the exterior syndrome due to wind-heat.

DIRECTIONS

To be taken orally, one pill each time, twice a day.

PRECAUTION

Not advised for the patients with the exterior syndrome of wind-cold.

003 LINGQIAO JIEDU WAN (羚翘解毒丸)

Antitoxic Pill of Antelope's Horn and Forsythia

PRINCIPAL INGREDIENTS

Antelope's horn (Cornu Antelopis), Honeysuckle flower (Flos Lonicerae), Arctium fruit (Fructus Arctii), Forsythia fruit (Fructus Forsythiae), Platycodon root

（Radix Platycodi）, Peppermint （Herba Menthae ）, Lophantherum （Herba Lophatheri）, Schizonepeta spike （Spica Schizonepetae）, Liquorice （Radix Glycyrrhizae）,Fermented soybean （Semen Sojiae Praeparata）

FUNCTION

Relieving the exterior syndrome with drugs pungent in flavor and cool in property, clearing away heat.

INDICATION

The onset of common cold of wind-heat type marked by fever, headache , cough, dry mouth and sore throat, red tip of the tongue with thin yellow fur, rapid pulse.

DIRECTIONS

To be taken orally, one to two pills each time, twice a day.

PRECAUTION

Spicy and greasy food should be avoided to take.

004   LINGYANG GANMAO PIAN （羚羊感冒片）

Tablet of Antelope's Horn for Common Cold

PRINCIPAL INGREDIENTS

Antelope's horn （Cornu Antelopis）, Forsythia fruit (Fructus Forsythiae), Honeysuckle flower （Flos Lonicerae）, Trichosanthes root （Radix Trichosanthis）, Platycodon root (Radix Platycodi), Pueraria root (Radix Puerariae)

FUNCTIONS

Dispelling wind, removing heat and inducing diaphoresis to reduce fever.

INDICATION

Influenza manifested as fever, headache, swelling and pain of throat, cough, dizziness, red tongue with thin and white or yellow coating and floating and rapid pulse. It is also used to treat redness and swelling of parotidis, etc.

DIRECTIONS

To be taken orally, four tablets each time, twice a day.

PRECAUTION

Spicy and greasy food should be avoided to take.

005 GANMAO QINGRE CHONGJI （感冒清热冲剂）

Infusion for Treating Coryza of Wind-Cold Type

PRINCIPAL INGREDIENTS

Schizonepeta spike (Spica Schizonepetae), Peppermint (Herba Menthae), Ledebouriella root (Radix Ledebouriellae), Perilla leaf (Folium Perillae), Bupleurum root (Radix Bupleuri), Pueraria root (Radix Puerariae), Platycodon root (Radix Platycodi), Bitter apricot seed (Semen Armeniacae Amarum), Dahurian angelica root (Radix Angelicae Dahuricae), Corydalis (Herba Corydalis Bungeanae), Reed rhizome (Rhizoma Phragmitis)

FUNCTIONS

Expelling wind and cold pathogens and inducing diaphoresis to reduce fever.

INDICATION

Common cold of wind-cold type, manifested as headache, fever, aversion to cold, pantalgia, watery nasal discharge, cough, dry throat, thin and white coating of the tongue and floating pulse.

DIRECTIONS

To be taken orally after being infused in boiling water, 12g each time, twice a day.

PRECAUTIONS

Spicy and greasy food should be avoided to take.

006 DOULIANG WAN （都梁丸）

Pill of Douliang

PRINCIPAL INGREDIENTS

Angelica dahurica root （Radix Angelicae Dahuricae）

FUNCTIONS

Dispelling wind and removing cold.

INDICATION

The women before and after child birth affected by wind- cold with the symptoms of fever, headache, dizziness, the tongue with thin and white coating and floating pulse. It is also used to treat common cold with the above symptoms

DIRECTIONS

To be taken orally, one to two pills each time, twice a day.

PRECAUTION

Spicy and greasy food should be avoided to take.

007 WUSHI CHA CHONGJI （午时茶冲剂）

Infusion of Noon Tea

PRINCIPAL INGREDIENTS

Angelica dahurica root （Radix Angelicae Dahuricae）, Wrinkled gianthyssop （Herba

Agastachis), Leaf of purple perilla (Folium Perillae), Pinellia tuber (Rhizoma Pinelliae), Tangerine peel (Perticarpium Citri Reticulatae), Magnolia bark (Cortex Magnoliae Officinalis), Root of balloon flower (Radix Platycodi), Prepared licorice root (Radix Glycyrrhizae Praeparata), Bupleurum root (Radix Bupleuri), Chuanxiong rhizome (Rhizoma Ligustici Chuanxiong), Fruit of citron or trifoliate orange (Fructus Aurantii), Notopterygium root (Rhizoma seu Radix Notopterygii), Platycodon root (Radix Platycodi), Peucedanum praeruptorum root (Radix Peucedani), Ledebouriella divaricata root (Radix Ledebouriellae)

FUNCTIONS

Dispelling wind and cold, promoting digestion and regulating the stomach.

INDICATION

Vomiting and diarrhea due to exterior cold-wind or retention of food due to improper diet marked by chills, fever, headache, fullness sensation and oppressed feeling in the chest and abdomen, vomiting, diarrhea, borborygmus and abdominal pain, white and greasy tongue fur and slippery pulse. The common cold of gastrointestinal type, influenza, acute gastroenteritis, etc. with the above symptoms can be used.

DIRECTIONS

To be taken orally ofter being infused in boiling water, 9g each time, twice a day.

PRECAUTION

Spicy and greasy food should be avoided to take.

008 YIN HUANG KOUFUYE (银黄口服液)

Oral Liquid of Honeysuckle Flower and Scutellaria

PRINCIPAL INGREDIENTS

Honeysuckle flower (Flos Lonicerae), Scutellaria root (Radix Scutellariae)

FUNCTIONS

Clearing away heat and toxic materials and relieving inflammation.

INDICATION

For the treatment of the common cold, acute tonsillitis, encephalitis B, epidemic cerebrospinal meningitis and infection of upper respiratory with the symptoms of fever, headache, cough, sore throat, red tongue with yellow fur, rapid pulse.

DIRECTIONS

To be taken orally, 10～20ml each time,

twice or three times a day.

PRECAUTION

Spicy and greast food should be avoided to take

009   HUOXIANG ZHANGQI WAN （藿香正气丸）

Pill of Agastache for Restoring Health

PRINCIPAL INGREDIENTS

Agastache rugosus herb （Herba Agastachis）, Shell of areca nut （Pericarpium Arecae）, Dahurian angelica root （Radix Angelicae Dahuricae）, Leaf of purple perilla （Folium Perillae）, Tuckahoe （Poria）, Pinellia tuber （Rhizoma Pinelliae）, Bighead atractylodes rhizome （Rhizoma Atractylodis Macrocephalae）, Tangerine peel （Perticarpium Citri Reticulatae）, Magnolia bark （Cortex Magnoliae Officinalis）, Root of balloon flower （Radix Platycodi）, Prepared licorice root （Radix Glycyrrhizae Praeparata）

FUNCTIONS

Relieving exterior syndrome, eliminating dampness and regulating Qi and the stomach.

INDICATION

Vomiting and diarrhea due to exterior cold

with interior dampness marked by chills, fever, headache, fullness sensation and oppressed feeling in the chest and abdomen, vomiting, diarrhea, borborygmus and abdominal pain, thick and greasy tongue fur, rapid pulse. The common cold of gastrointestinal type, influenza, acute gastroenteritis, gastroduodenal ulcer, chronic colitis, food poisoning, epidemic parotitis and other diseases belonging to exterior cold with endogenous dampness can be treated with the drug.

DIRECTIONS

To be taken orally, one pill each time, twice a day.

PRECAUTION

Spicy and greasy food should be avoided to take.

010 XIAOCHAIHU WAN（小柴胡丸）

Minor Pill of Bupleurum

PRINCIPAL INGREDIENTS

Bupleurum root (Radix Bupleuri), Scutellaria root (Radix Scutellariae), Pinellia tuber (Rhizoma Pinelliae), Fresh ginger (Rhizoma Zingiberis Recens), Ginseng (Radix Ginseng), Chinese date (Fructus Ziziphi Jujubae), Prepared licorice root (Radix Glycyrrhizae Praeparata)

FUNCTIONS

Treating shaoyang disease by mediation.

INDICATION

Shaoyang disease with the pathogenic factors located neither in the exterior nor in the interior but in between them marked by alternate attacks of chills and fever, fullness in the chest, hypochondriac discomfort, anorexia, dysphasia, retching, bitterness in the mouth, dry throat, dizziness, thin and white fur of the tongue and stringy pulse, or exogenous febrile diseases occurring in women belonging to invasion of the blood chamber by pathogenic heat. The common cold, malaria, infection of biliary tract, hepatitis, pleuritis, chronic gastritis, mastosis, intercostal neuralgia manifested with the above symptoms can be treated with the drug.

DIRECTIONS

To be taken orally, one pill each time, twice a day.

PRECAUTION

Patients with syndromes such as upper excess with lower deficiency, or excess of liver-fire, hyperactivity of the liver-Yang, haematomesis due to deficiency of Yin are forbidden to use the drug.

011 FANGFENG TONGSHENG WAN（防风通圣丸）

Miraculous Pill of Ledebouriella

PRINCIPAL INGREDIENTS

Ledebouriella root (Radix Ledebouriellae), Shizonepeta spike (Spica Shizonepetae), Peppermint (Herba Menthae), Rhubarb (Radix et Rhizoma Rhei), Mirabilite (Natrii Sulphas), Capejasmine fruit (Fructus Gardeniae), Platycodon root (Radix Platycodi), Gypsum (Gypsum Fibrosum), Chuanxiong rhizome (Rhizoma Ligustici Chuanxiong), Chinese angelica root (Radix Angelicae Sinensis), White peony root (Radix Paeoniae Alba), Scutellaria root (Radix Scutellariae), Forsythia fruit (Fructus Forsythiae), Liquorice (Radix Glycyrrhizae), Bighead atractylodes rhizome (Rhizoma Atractylodis Macrocephalae)

FUNCTIONS

Relieving exterior syndrome, removing obstruction due to interior syndrome, clearing away heat and toxic materials.

INDICATION

Wind-heat in the exterior and dampness-heat in the interior, marked by excess of both interior and exterior, manifested as chilliness, high fever, headache, dry throat, constipation, dark urine, or the primary symptoms of boils eczema and itching, thick and greasy tongue fur, rapid pulse.

DIRECTIONS

To be taken orally, 6g each time, twice a day.

PRECAUTION

It should be used cautiously for patients in pregnancy.

012 QINGXUAN PIAN（清眩片）

Tablet for Relieving Dizziness

PRINCIPAL INGREDIENTS

Angelica dahurica root（Radix Angelicae Dahuricae）, Chuanxiong rhizome（Rhizoma Ligustici Chuanxiong）, Schizonepeta tenuifolia herb（Herba Schizonepetae）, Gypsum（Gypsum Fibrosum）, Field mint or Chinese peppermint herb（Herba Menthae）

FUNCTIONS

Dispelling wind and heat, relieving pain and dizziness.

INDICATION

Headache and dizziness due to wind-heat, companioned with the symptoms of swelling and pain of throat, cough, fullness sensation in the abdomen, vomiting, red tongue with yellow coating and floating and rapid pulse.

DIRECTIONS

To be taken orally, 4~6 tablets each time, twice a day.

PRECAUTION

Spicy and greasy food should be avoided to take.

013 XIONGJU SHANGQING WAN （芎菊上清丸）

Pill of Chuanxiong and Chrysanthemum for Clearing Upper Heat

PRINCIPAL INGREDIENTS

Chuanxiong rhizome (Rhizoma Ligustici Chuanxiong), Chrysanthemum flower (Flos Chrysanthemii), Peppermint (Herba Menthae), Forsythia fruit (Fructus Forsythiae), Schizonepeta (Herba Schizonepetae), Ledebouriella root (Radix Ledebouriellae), Dahurian angelica root (Radix Angelicae Dahuriae), Scutellaria root (Radix Scutel-

lariae), Phellodendron bark (Cortex Phellodendri), Capejasmine fruit (Fructus Gardeniae),Rhubarb (Radix et Rhizoma Rhei),
Platycodon root (Radix Platycodi)

FUNCTIONS

Expelling wind and heat, purging pathogenic fire and relaxing the bowels.

INDICATION

The attack of pathogenic wind-heat on the
upper and middle parts of the body marked
by dizziness, tinnitus, dry nose and eyes,
oral ulceration, swelling and pain in the
gums and constipation, red tongue with yellow coating and floating and rapid pulse.

DIRECTIONS

To be taken orally, one pill each time,
twice a day.

PRECAUTION

Not advisable for pregnant women. Spicy
and greasy food should be avoided to take.

014 JINFANG BAIDU WAN （荆防败毒丸）

Antiphlogistic Pill of Schizonepeta and
Ledebourielea

PRINCIPAL INGREDIENTS

Schizonepata tenuifolia herb （ Herba
Schizonepatae）, Ledebouriela root （Radix

Ledebourielae）, Bupleurum root （Radix Bupleuri）, Peucedanum root （Radix Peucedani）, Chuanxiong rhizome （Rhizoma Ligustici Chuanxiong）, Citron or trifoliate orange fruit （Fructus Aurantii）, Notopterygium root （Rhizoma seu Radix Notopterygii）, Pubescent angelica root （Radix Angelicae Pubescentis）, Poria （Poria）, Platycodon root （Radix Platycodi）

FUNCTIONS

Expelling wind to relieve exterior symptoms, Removing noxious heat and relieving swelling.

INDICATION

The onset of common cold of wind-cold type and The onset of furunculosis marked by chill, fever, headache, the tongue with thin white fur, superficial pulse.

DIRECTIONS

To be taken orally, one pill each time, twice a day.

PRECAUTION

Spicy and greasy food should be avoided to take.

015 SHENSU WAN （参苏丸）

Pill of Ginseng and Perilla

PRINCIPAL INGREDIENTS

Ginseng (Radix Ginseng), Perilla leaf (Folium Perillae), Peraria root (Radix Pureariae), Platycodon root (Radix Platycodi), Purple-flowered peucedanum root (Radix Peucedani Peucedanum), Fruit of citron or trifoliate orange (Fructus Aurantii), Poria (Poria), Licorice root (Radix Glycyrrhizae), Aucklandia root (Radix Aucklandiae), Tangerine peel (Pericarpium Citri Rediculatae), Pinellia tuber (Rhizoma Pinelliae)

FUNCTIONS

Tonifying Qi and expelling wind to relieve exterior symptoms, moistening the lung to resolve phlegm.

INDICATION

Exopathic disease caused by weakened body resistance and pathogenic wind-cold-dampness, such as common cold, influenza and bronchitis, etc. manifested as chill, fever headache, stuffy nose, cough and plenty phlegm, fullness and stuffiness in the chest, white and greasy coating of the tongue, floating and soft pulse.

DIRECTIONS

To be taken orally, one pill each time,

twice a day.

PRECAUTION

Spicy and greasy food should be avoided to take.

016 YUPINGFENG WAN （玉屏风丸）

Jade-Screen Pill

PRINCIPAL INGREDIENTS

Ledebouriella root (Radix Ledebouriellae), Astragalus root (Radix Astragali seu Hedysari), Bighead atractylodes rhizome (Rhizoma Atractylodis Macrocephalae)

FUNCTIONS

Invigorating Qi and consolidating the superficial resistance to arrest perspiration.

INDICATION

Failure of superficial-Qi to protect the body against diseases marked by spontaneous perspiration, excessive sweating, liability to wind pathogen, pale complexion, pale tongue with white fur, and floating , feeble and soft pulse. Hyperhidrosis, allergic rhinitis , chronic rhinitis and susceptibility to the common cold manifested as failure of superficial-Qi to protect the body against diseases can be treated with the drug.

DIRECTIONS

To be taken orally, one pill each time, twice a day.

PRECAUTION

The drug is contraindicated in patients with night sweat due to interior heat caused by deficiency of Yin.

017 CHAIHU YIN CHONGJI （柴胡饮冲剂）

Infusion of Bupleurum Yin

PRINCIPAL INGREDIENTS

Bulpeurum root (Radix Bupleuri), Ginseng (Radix Ginseng), Scutellaria root (Radix Scutellariae), Licorice root (Radix Glycyrrhizae), Peony root (Radix Paeoniae), Platycodon root (Radix Pyatycodi), Pinellia tuber (Rhizoma Pinelliae), Chinese angelica root (Radix Angelicae Sinensis), Rhubarb root (Radix et Rhizoma Rhei), Schisandra fruit (Fructus Schisandrae)

FUNCTIONS

Strengthening the body resistance to expel pathogenic factors.

INDICATION

Because of weakened body resistance, the pathogenic factors passing through from the exterior to interior, such as common cold, TB, and infection of biliary tract, etc. manifested as alternate attacks of chill and fever, fullness in the chest and plenty phlegm, emaciation, sensation of heat felt in the chest, the palms and soles, dry mouth and throat, red tongue with reduced saliva, thready and feeble pulse.

DIRECTIONS

To be taken orally after being infused in boiling water, one packets each time, three times a day.

PRECAUTION

Spicy and greasy food should be avoided to take.

018 CHUANXIONG CHATIAO KOUFUYE
（川芎茶调口服液）

Oral Liquid of Chuanxiong Mixture

PRINCIPAL INGREDIENTS

Chuanxiong rhizome (Rhizoma Ligustici Chuanxiong), Schizonepeta (Herba Schizonepetae), Dahurian angelica root (Radix Angelicae Dahuricae), Notopterygium root (Rhizoma seu Radix Notopterygii), Licorice root (Radix Glycyrrhizae), Wild ginger (Herba Asari), Ledebouriella root (radix Ledebouriellae), Peppermint (Herba Menthae)

FUNCTIONS

Dispelling exopathic wind to relieve pain.

INDICATION

Common cold, migraine, nervous headache, headache due to chronic rhinitis marked by attacking of exopathic wind manifested with the symptoms of headache, migraine, or pain on the top of head, aversion to cold with fever, obstruction of nose, dizziness, thin and white fur of the tongue, floating and slippery pulse.

DIRECTIONS

To be taken orally, one pill each time, twice a day.

PRECAUTION

Spicy and greasy food should be avoided to take.

019　GANMAO TUIRE CHONGJI（感冒退热冲剂）

Cold-Fever-Treating Infusion

PRINCIPAL INGREDIENTS

Isatis leaf (Folium Isatidis), Isatis root (Radix Isatidis), Forsythia fruit (Fructus Forsythiae), Rhizoma of bistort (Rhizoma Bistortae)

FUNCTIONS

Clearing away heat and toxic materials.

INDICATION

Upper respiratory tract infection, acute tonsillitis and laryngopharyngitis with the symptoms of fever, headache, obstruction of nose, thin and yellow fur of the tongue, floating and rapid pulse.

DIRECTIONS

To be taken orally after being infused in boiling water each time, three times a day.

PRECAUTION

Avoid raw, cold and greasy food.

020 CHAIHU ZHUSHEYE (柴胡注射液)

Injection of Bulpeurum

PRINCIPAL INGREDIENTS

Bulpeurum root (Radix Bupleuri)

FUNCTIONS

Reducing fever.

INDICATION

Common cold, influenza and other diseases with high fever can be used the drug to reduce fever as an assistant treatment drug.

DIRECTIONS

Intramuscular injection, 24ml each time, 12 times each day. The dosage should be reduced for children.

021 BANNANGEN CHONGJI （板蓝根冲剂）

Infusion of Isatis Root

PRINCIPAL INGREDIENTS

Isatis root (Radix Isatidis), Isatis leaf (Folium Isatidis)

FUNCTIONS

Clearing away heat and toxic materials, cooling blood and subduing swelling.

INDICATION

Influenza and common cold manifested as headache, fever, swollen and sore throat and cough. It can also be used to prevent epidemic encephalitis B.

DIRECTIONS

To be taken orally after being infused in boiling water, one packet each time, three times a day.

PRECAUTION

Avoid raw, cold and greasy food.

022 MEISU WAN （梅苏丸）

Pill of Japanese Apricot and Perilla Leaf

PRINCIPAL INGREDIENTS

Japanese Apricot fruit (Fructus Mume), Perilla Leaf (Folium Perillae), Herb of field mint or Chinese peppermint (Herba Men-

thae）, Oil of field mint or Chinese peppermint herb (Oleum Herba Menthae)

FUNCTIONS

Clearing away summer-heat.

INDICATION

Common cold in the summer, sunstroke,
heat stroke with the symptoms of fever,
profuse perspiration, restlessness, thirst,
dark urine, thin and yellow fur of the
tongue, floating, feeble and rapid pulse.

DIRECTIONS

To be taken orally, five pills each time,
three times a day.

PRECAUTION

Auoid raw, cold and greasy food.

023　BAOJI WAN（保济丸）

Health Pill

PRINCIPAL INGREDIENTS

Gastrodia tuber (Rhizoma Gastrodiae),
Dahurian angelica rootastrodia tuber (Rhi-
zoma Gastrodiae), Dahurian angelica root
（Radix Angelicae Dahuricae）, Aucklandia
root (Radix Aucklandiae), Cablin pacholi
（Herba Pogostemonis）, Magnolia Bark
（Cortex Magnoliae Officinalis）, Atracty-
lodes rhizome (Rhizoma Atracylodis)

FUNCTIONS

Relieving pain by regulating Qi, relieving exterior syndrome and eliminating dampness.

INDICATION

Common cold in the four seasons, abdominal pain, vomiting, diarrhea , discomfort in the stomach and intestines, indigestion, white coating of the tongue, floating and soft pulse.

DIRECTIONS

To be taken orally, 2~4g each time, three times a day.

PRECAUTION

Spicy and greasy food should be avoided to take.

024   TIANJIN GANMAO PIAN（天津感冒片）

Tianjin Cold-Treating Tablet

PRINCIPAL INGREDIENTS

Arctium fruit (Fructus Arctii), Platycodon root (Radix Platycodi), Forsythia fruit (Fructus Forsythiae), Honeysuckle flower (Flos Lonicerae), Prepared soybean (Semen Sojae Preparata)

FUNCTIONS

Clearing away pathogenic heat and wind,

relieving exterior syndrome and reducing
fever.

INDICATION

Influenza and common cold with the symptoms of chill and fever, distress of limbs,
headache, cough, swollen and pain of
throat. red tongue with thin white or yellow fur, rapid pulse.

DIRECTIONS

To be taken orally, 3~6 tablets each time,
three times a day.

PRECAUTION

Avoid raw, cold and greasy food.

I −2 Prescriptions for Heat-clearing
清热剂

025 QINGWEN JIEDU WAN （清瘟解毒丸）

Antipyretic and Antitoxic Pill

PRINCIPAL INGREDIENTS

Isatis leaf (Folium Isatidis), Forsythia fruit
(Fructus Forsythiae), Scrophularia root
(Radix Scrophulariae), Trichosanthes root
(Radix Trichosanthis), Platycodon root
(Radix Platycodi), Arctium fruit (parched)
(Fructus Arctii), Notopterygium root
(radix seu Rhizoma Notopterygii),Dahurian

angelica root (Radix Angelicae Dahuricae),
Ledebouriella root (Radix Ledebouriellae),
Pueraria root (Radix Puerariae), Bupleurum
root (Radix Bupleuri), Scutellaria root
(Radix Scutellariae), Chuanxiong rhizome
(Rhizoma Ligustici Chuanxiong), Red pe-
ony root (Radix Paeoniae Rubra), Liquorice
(Radix Glycyrrhizae), Lophatherum (Herba
Lophatheri)

FUNCTIONS
Having antipyretic and antitoxin function.

INDICATION
Influenza, marked by fever with chills an-
hidrosis with headache, thirst and dry
throat, aching pain of limbs, red tongue
with yellow fur, rapid pulse. It is also used
to treat swelling and pain of mumps.

DIRECTIONS
To be taken orally, one pill each time,
twice a day. For children, the doses should
be correspondingly reduced.

PRECAUTION
Spicy and greasy food should be avoided to
take.

026 NIUHUANG JIEDU WAN （牛黄解毒丸）
Cow-Bezoar Antitoxic Pill

PRINCIPAL INGREDIENTS

Cow-bezoar (Calculus Bovis), Realgar (Realgar), Gypsum (Gypsum Fibrosum), Borneol (Borneolum), Rhubarb (Radix et Rhizoma Rhei), Scutellaria root (Radix Scutellariae), Platycodon root (Radix Platycodi), Liquorice (Radix Glycyrrhizae)

FUNCTIONS

Clearing away heat and toxic materials.

INDICATION

The internal excess of pathogenic fire and heat marked by swelling pain of the throat and gingival, oral ulceration, conjunctiva congestion, swelling and pain of the eyes and so on, red tongue with yellow coating, rapid pules.

DIRECTIONS

To be taken orally, one pill each time, twice to three times a day.

PRECAUTION

Spicy and greasy food should be avoided to take, Contraindicated for women in pregnancy.

027　XIHUANG WAN（犀黄丸）

Pill of Cow-Bezoar

PRINCIPAL INGREDIENTS

Artificial cow-bezoar (Calculus Bovis Fracticius), Musk (Moschus), Frankincense (Resina Olibani), Myrrh (Myrrha)

FUNCTIONS

Detoxicating and resolving masses, subduing swelling and alleviating pain.

INDICATION

Carbuncle and boils, multiple abscesses, lymphnoditis, cold abscess, lung cancer, red tongue with yellow coating, rapid pules.

DIRECTIONS

To be taken orally, 3g pill each time, twice a day.

PRECAUTION

Contraindicated for patients in pregnant. Spicy and greasy food should be avoided to take.

028 HUANGLIAN SHANGQING WAN （黄连上清丸）

Pill of Coptis for Dispelling Upper Heat

PRINCIPAL INGREDIENTS

Coptis root (Rhizoma Coptidis), Scutellaria (Radix Scutellariae), Rhubarb (Radix and Rhizoma Rhei), Phellodendrom bark (Cortex Phellodendri), Gypsum (Gypsum Fibrosum), Forsythia fruit (Fructus Forsythiae), Chuanxiong rhizome (Rhizoma Ligustici Chuanxiong), Chrysanthemum flower (Flos Chrysanthemi), Dahurian angelica root (Radix Angelicae Dahuricae), Peppermint (Herba Menthae), Platycodon root (Radix Platycodi), Schizonepeta spike (Spica Schizonepetae)

FUNCTIONS

Dispersing pathogenic wind, relieving pain, clearing away heat and loosening the bowels.

INDICATION

The attack of wind-heat on the upper and middle parts of the human body, manifested as dizziness, headache, conjunctiva congestion and swelling, toothache, aphthae, constipation, scanty dark urine, red tongue with yellow coating, rapid pules.

DIRECTIONS

To be taken orally, two pills each time, twice a day.

PRECAUTION

Never administrated to pregnant women.

029 HUANGLIAN QINGWEI WAN (黄连清胃丸)

Pill of Coptis for Dispelling Heat in Stomach

PRINCIPAL INGREDIENTS

Coptis root (Rhizoma Coptidis), Forsythia fruit (Fructus Forsythiae), Rhubarb (Radix and Rhizoma Rhei), Phellodendron bark (Cortex Phellodendri), Tangerine peel (Pericarpium Citri Reticulatae)

FUNCTIONS

Clearing stomach-heat, relieving inflammation.

INDICATION

Stagnation of heat in the stomach marked by headache radiated by toothache, feverish cheeks, aversion to heat with predilection for cold, ulceration in the gum, or swelling and soreness of the tongue, lips and cheeks, red tongue with yellow coating, slippery strong and rapid pulse. It can be used to deal with periodontitis, stomatitis, gingival pustular swelling, etc.

DIRECTIONS

To be taken orally, one pill each time, twice a day.

PRECAUTION

It is not fit for the patients with deficiency syndrome. Spicy and greasy food should be avoided to take.

030   LIANGGE SAN （凉膈散）

Powder for Cooling Diaphragm

PRINCIPAL INGREDIENTS

Rhubarb （Radix et Rhizoma Rhei）, Mirabilite （Natrii）, Liquorice root （Radix Glycyrrhizae）, Capejasmine fruit （Fructus Gardeniae）, Skutellaria root （Radix Scutellariae）, Forsythia fruit （Fructus Forsythiae）, Herb of field mint or Chinese peppermint （Herba Menthae）

FUNCTIONS

Purging pathogenic heat accumulated in diaphragm.

INDICATION

Infectious or non-infectious febrile diseases with the symptoms of high fever or tidal fever, delirium, headache, sore throat, constipation, distention and fullness in the chest and abdomen, hot and dark urine, red tongue with yellow coating, rapid pulse.

DIRECTIONS

To be taken orally, 6g each time, twice a day.

PRECAUTION

The administration is prohibited or should

be careful for those with weak constitution and in pregnant. Spicy and greasy food should be avoided to take.

031 NIUHUANG SHANGQING WAN (牛黄上清丸)

Cow-Bezoar Pill for Clearing Upper Heat

PRINCIPAL INGREDIENTS

Cow-bezoar (calculus Bovis), Peppermint (Herba Menthae), Chrysanthemum flower (Flos Chrysanthemi), Schizonepeta spike (Spice Schizonepetae), Dahurian angelica root (Radix Angelicae Dahuricae), Chuanxiong rhizome (Rhizoma Ligustici Chuanxiong), Capejasmine fruit (Fructus Gardeniae), Coptis root (Rhizoma Coptidis), Phellodendron bark (Cortex Phellodendri), Scutellaria root (Radix Scutellariae), Rhubarb root (Radix et Rhizoma Rhei), Forsythia fruit (Fructus Forsythiae), Red peony root (Radix Paeoniae Rubra), Chinese angelica root (Radix Angelicae Sinensis), Rehmannia root (Radix Rehmanniae), Platycodon root (Radix Platycodi), Gypsum (Gypsum Fibrosum), Borneol (Borneolum), Liquorice (Radix Glycyrrhizae)

FUNCTIONS

Clearing away heat and purging pathogenic fire, dispelling wind and relieving pain.

INDICATION

The syndromes of excessive fire in the middle and upper parts of the human body or the attack of pathogenic wind and heat on the upper part of the body marked by headache, vertigo, conjunctiva congestion, tinnitus swelling and sore throat, ulcerations of mouth and tongue, swelling and soreness of the gums, constipation and dry stool, red tongue with yellow coating, rapid pules.

DIRECTIONS

To be taken orally, one pill each time, twice a day.

PRECAUTION

Pregnant women should be careful when taking this medicine.

032 GANLU XIAODU DAN （甘露消毒丹）

Pill of Ganlu for Disinfecting

PRINCIPAL INGREDIENTS

Talc (Talcum), Scutellaria (Radix Scutellariae), Oriental wormwood (Herba Artemisiae), Wrinkled giant hyssop (Herba

Agastachis), Forsythia fruit (Fructus Forsythiae), Grass-leafed sweet flag rhizome (Rhizoma Acori Graminei), Herb of field mint or Chinese peppermint (Herba Menthae),Round cardamon seed (Semen Amoni Cardamoni), Blackberry lily rhizome (Rhizoma Belamandae), Tendril-leaf fritillary bulb (Bulbus Fritillarie Cirrhosae), Clematis armandii stem (Caulis Clematidis Armandii), Liquorice root (Radix Glycyrrhizae)

FUNCTIONS

Clearing away pathogenic fire and toxic material, removing dampness and heat.

INDICATION

Influenza, acute infectious hepatitis, acute gastroenteritis, bacillary dysentery, etc. with the syndromes of fire-dampness manifested as intense heat, dysentery with fever, dizziness, conjunctival congestion, otalgia, tinnitus, hypochondriac pain, bitter taste, dark urine, jaundice, red tongue with yellow and greasy coating, rapid pules.

DIRECTIONS

To be taken orally, 9g each time, twice a day.

PRECAUTION

Spicy and greasy food should be avoided to take.

033 ZHONGMAN FENXIAO WAN (中满分消丸)

Pill for Relieving the Fullness in the Abdomen

PRINCIPAL INGREDIENTS

Ginseng (Radix Ginseng), Bighead atractylodes rhizome (Rhizoma Atractylodis Macrocephalae), Poria (Poria), Liquorice root (Radix Glycyrrhizae), Tangerine peel (Pericarpium Citri Reticulatae), Amomum fruit (Fructus Amomi), Coptis root (Rhizoma Coptidis), Scutellaria root (Radix Scutellariae), Oriental water plantain (Rhizoma Alismatis), Magnolia bark (Cortex Magnoliae Officinalis), Immature bitter orange (Fructus Aurantii Immaturus), Pinellia tuber (Rhizoma Pinelliae), Ginger rhizome (Rhizoma Zingiberis), Anemarrhena rhizome (Rhizoma Anemarrhenae), Common turmeric rhizome (Rhizoma Curcumae Longae), Umbellate pore fungus (Polyporus Umbellatus)

FUNCTIONS

Strengthening the spleen and regulating Qi,

clearing away pathogenic fire and removing dampness.

INDICATION

The patients with spleen deficiency and heat- dampness syndromes manifested as fullness sensation and oppressed feeling in the abdomen, bitter taste, nausea, constipation, dark urine, red tongue with yellow and greasy coating, rapid pules.

DIRECTIONS

To be taken orally, one pill each time, twice a day.

PRECAUTION

Spicy and greasy food should be avoided to take.

034 LONGDAN XIEGAN WAN （龙胆泻肝丸）
Pill of Gentian for Purring Liver-Fire

PRINCIPAL INGREDIENTS

Gentian root (Radix Gentianae), Bupleurum root (Radix Bupleuri), Scutellaria root (Radix Scutellariae), Capejasmine fruit (Fructus Gardeniae), Oriental water plantain rhizome (Rhizoma Alismatis), Akebia stem (Caulis Akebiae), Plantain seed (Semen Plantaginis), Chinese Angelica root (Radix Angelicae Sinensis), Rehmannia root

(Radix Rehmanniae), Liquorice root (Radix Glycyrrhizae)

FUNCTIONS

Clearing away pathogenic fire in the liver and gallbladder, removing dampness and heat.

INDICATION

The fire of excess type or dampness-heat in the liver and gallbladder manifested as dizziness, conjunctival congestion, otalgia, tinnitus, hypochondriac pain, bitter taste, dark urine, difficulty and pain in micturition, red tongue with yellow and greasy coating, rapid pules.

DIRECTIONS

To be taken orally, 9g each time, twice a day.

PRECAUTION

Spicy and greasy food should be avoided to take. It should be given to pregnant women with great care.

035 DANGGUI LONGHUI WAN (当归龙荟丸)

Pill of Angelica, Gentian and Aloes

PRINCIPAL INGREDIENTS

Chinese angelica root (Radix Angelicae Sinensis), Gentian root (Radix Gentianae),

Aloes （Aloe）, Scutellaria root （Radix Scutellariae）, Coptis Rhizome （Rhizoma Coptidis）, Phellodendron bark （Cortex Phellodendri）, Capejasmine fruit （Fructus Gardeniae）, Rhubarb （Radix and Rhizoma Rhei）, Aucklandia root （Radix Aucklandiae）, Musk （Moschus）

FUNCTIONS

Clearing away pathogenic fire in the liver and gallbladder.

INDICATION

The fire of excess heat type in the liver and gallbladder manifested as headache, dizziness, conjunctival congestion, deafness, pain and bulge of ear, hypochondriac pain, bitter taste, dark urine, constipation, red tongue with yellow coating, rapid pules.

DIRECTIONS

To be taken orally, one pill each time, twice a day.

PRECAUTION

Spicy and greasy food should be avoided to take.

036   DAIGE SAN （黛蛤散）

Powder of Indigo and Clam Shell

PRINCIPAL INGREDIENTS

Natural indigo （Indiga Naturalis）, Clam Shell （Concha Meretricis seu Cyclinae）

FUNCTIONS

Purging pathogenic heat accumulated in the lung and removing phlegm to relieve cough.

INDICATION

Cough with profuse sputum due to lung-heat, reddened tongue with yellow coating and fine rapid pulse. It can be used to treat bronchitis.

DIRECTIONS

To be taken orally, 6-9g each time, twice a day.

PRECAUTION

Spicy and greasy food should be avoided to take.

037 **XIAKUCAO GAO** （夏枯草膏）

Semifluid Extract of Prunella

PRINCIPAL INGREDIENTS

Fruit-spike of common selfheal （Spica Prunellae）

FUNCTIONS

Clearing away heat, removing phlegm and relieving swelling.

INDICATION

Thyroid enlargement, lymphaden hypertrophy, tuberculous lymphadenitis, lobuli hyperplasia, hypertension marked with dizziness, red tongue with yellow fur, rapid pulse

DIRECTIONS

To be taken orally, 10g each time, three times a day.

PRECAUTION

Spicy and greasy food should be avoided to take.

038 PIANZIHUANG （片仔癀）

Anti-Inflammatory and Analgesic Bolus

PRINCIPAL INGREDIENTS

Not yet published.

FUNCTIONS

Clearing away heat and toxic materials, relieving swelling and pain.

INDICATION

Acute or chronic hepatitis, tympanitis, gum abscess, oral ulcer, bee sting, snakebite, nail-like boil and innominate inflammatory swelling.

DIRECTIONS

To be taken orally, children 1~8 years, 0. 15~0. 3g; over 8 years and adults 0. 6g each time. All twice to three times a day.

Spicy and greasy food should be avoided to take.

039 XINHUANG PIAN （新癀片） *

New Type Tablet of Anti-Inflammatory and Analgesics

PRINCIPAL INGREDIENTS

Cow-bezoar (Calculus Bovis), Pearl (Margarita), Notoginseng root (Radix Notoginseng)

FUNCTIONS

Clearing away heat and toxic materials, relieving selling and pain, anti-inflammation.

INDICATION

Acute hepatitis, tympanitis, rheumatic arthritis, cholecystitis, inflammatory swelling, etc. marked with fever, or jaundice, or swelling and pain, red tongue with yellow coating and rapid pulse.

DIRECTIONS

To be taken orally, 2～4 tablets each time, three times a day; To betaken externally, added water to soft it then applying it to affected area.

PRECAUTION

It should be used with care by pregnant

women. Spicy and greasy food should be avoided to take.

040   LIU YING WAN （六应丸）

Anti-Inflammatory Pill

PRINCIPAL INGREDIENTS

Pearl （Margarita）, Cow-bezoar （Calculus Bovis）, Toad venom （Venenum Bufonis）

FUNCTIONS

Clearing away heat and toxic material, subduing swelling and pain.

INDICATION

Tonsillitis, furuncle, sore, diseases of throat, the bite of insects, etc.

DIRECTIONS

To be taken orally, with boiled water. Adults 10 pills each time; children 5 pills each time; infants 2 pills each time, three times a day. For external use, disintegrate some pills in just a little cold boiled water of vinegar and then apply it to the affected part of skin.

PRECAUTION

Never to be administered to pregnant women.

041   BAZHENG HEJI （八正合剂）

Liquid of Eight Health Restoring

PRINCIPAL INGREDIENTS

Plantain seed (Semen Plantagini), Chinese pink herb (Herba Dianthi), Prostrate Knotweed (Herba Polygoni Avicularis), Tale (Talcum), Capejasmine fruit (Fructus Gardeniae), Prepared licorice root (Radix Glycyrrhizae Praeparata), Fiveleaf akebia (Caulis Akebiae), Rhubarb (Radix et Rhizoma Rhei), Rush pith (Medulla Junci)

FUNCTIONS

Clearing away heat and purging fire, inducing diuresis for treating stranguria.

INDICATION

Acute urethritis, cystitis, pyelitis, stone or infection in urinary system marked by stranguria due to dampness and heat manifested with the symptoms of subjective sensation of spasmodic distention and fullness of the lower abdomen, distending pain in the loin and abdomen, dribbling urination, difficulty in micturition or retention of urine, dryness of mouth and throat, red tongue with yellow fur and slippery forceful pulse.

DIRECTIONS

To be taken orally, 15～20ml each time, three times a day.

It is contraindicated in the debilitated and in pregnant. Spicy and greasy food should be avoided to take.

042 QIANLIETONG PIAN （前列通片）

Tablet for Treating Prostatitis and Prostatomegaly

PRINCIPAL INGREDIENTS

Astragalus root （Radix Astragali seu Hedysari）, Cinnamon bark （Cortex Cinnamomi）, Phellodendron bark （Cortex Phellodendri）, Amber （Succinum）, Plantain herb （Herba Plantaginis）, Dandelion herb （Herba Taraxaci）, Lycopus herb （Herba Lycopi）

FUNCTIONS

Tonifying kidney and spleen, clearing away dampness, promoting blood circulation to remove stasis.

INDICATION

Prostatitis and prostatomegaly marked by dribbling urination, difficulty in micturition, frequent and urgent micturition, retention of urine, pale or red tongue with white or yellow fur, slippery pulse.

DIRECTIONS

To be taken orally, 4~6 tablets each time, three times a day.

PRECAUTION

Spicy and greasy food should be avoided to take.

043 YINCHEN WULING WAN （茵陈五苓丸）
Pill of Wormwood and Five Drugs with Poria

PRINCIPAL INGREDIENTS

Oriental wormwood （Herba Artemisiae Capillaris）, Umbellate pore fungus （Polyporus Umbellatus）, Oriental water plantain rhizome （Rhizoma Alismatis）, Bighead atractylodes rhizome （Rhizoma Atractylodis Macrocephalae）, Poria （Poria）, Skullcap root （Radix Scutellariae）, Fruit of immature citron （Fructus Aurantii Immaturus）, Rhizome of Atractylodes lancea （Rhizoma Atractylodis）, Tangerine peel （Pericarpium Citri Reticulatae）, Medicated leaven （Massa Fermentata Medicinalis）, Licorice root （Radix Glycyrrhizae）, Hawthorn fruit （Fructus Crataegi）

FUNCTIONS

Clearing away heat and eliminating dampness to treat jaundice, strengthening the spleen and promoting Qi circulation, Promoting dissection to remove stagnated food.

INDICATION

Jaundice of acute infectious icterichepatitis, cholecystitis and colelithiasis characterized by bright yellow coloration of the skin and eyes, fullness sensation in the abdomen, disturbance in urination, yellow and greasy tongue fur, rapid and slippery pulse. Dysentery and diarrhea and indigestion, gastroenteritis, bacterial diarrhea as well as retention of acute urethritis, cystitis and pyelitis can be used with this drug.

DIRECTIONS

To be taken orally, 10g each time, three times a day.

PRECAUTION

Spicy and greasy food should be avoided to take. It should be careful to be used in pregnant women.

044 DANLE PIAN (胆乐片)

Tablet for Gall Pleased

PRINCIPAL INGREDIENTS

Bupleurum root (Radix Bupleuri), Oriental wormwood (Herba Artemisiae Capillaris), Capejasmine fruit (Fructus Gardeniae),

Rhubarb (Radix et Rhizoma Rhei), Curcuma root (Radix Curcumae), Cow-Bezoar (Calculus Bovis), Mongolian dandelion herb (Herba Taraxaci), Oil of field mint or Chinese peppermint herb (Oleum Herba Menthae)

FUNCTIONS

Clearing away heat and removing dampness, normalizing the function of the gall-bladder and removing calculi, soothing the liver and relieving pain, treating jaundice.

INDICATION

Cholecystitis and cholelithiasis with the symptoms of jaundice, fever and chill, fullness and pain in the chest, vomiting and nausea, red tongue with yellow and greasy fur, taut and rapid plus.

DIRECTIONS

To be taken orally, 4~5 tablets each time, three times a day.

PRECAUTION

Spicy and greasy food should be avoided to take. It should be careful for pregnant women.

045 LIDAN PAISHI CHONGJI （利胆排石冲剂）

Infusion of Cholagogic and Lithagogue

PRINCIPAL INGREDIENTS

Lysimachia (Herba Lysimachiae), Oriental wormwood (Herba Artemisiae Capillaris), Gentian root (Radix Gentianae), Bupleurum root (Radix Bupleuri), Curcuma root (Radix Curcumae), Rhubarb (Radix et Rhizoma Rhei), Mirabilite (Natrii Sulphas), Red peony root (Radix Paeoniae Rubra), Cattial Pollen (Pollen Typhae), Trogopterus Dung (Faeces Trogopterorum)

FUNCTIONS

Clearing away heat and removing dampness, normalizing the function of the gallbladder and removing calculi.

INDICATION

Biliary calculi, infection of biliary tract and cholecystitis manifested as dizziness, conjunctival congestion, otalgia, tinnitus, hypochondriac pain, bitter taste, dark urine, difficulty and pain in micturition.

DIRECTIONS

To be taken orally, 10g each time, twice a day.

PRECAUTION

Spicy and greasy food should be avoided to take. It is not administrated to pregnant.

046 JIUWEI QIANGHUO WAN（九味羌活丸）

Pill of Nine Components of Notopterygium

PRINCIPAL INGREDIENTS

Notopterygium root （Rhizoma seu Radix Notopterygii）, Ledebouriella root （Radix Ledebouriellae ）, Atractylodes rhizome （ Rhizoma Atractylodis ）, Asarum herb (Herba Asari）, Chuanxiong rhizome （Rhizoma Ligustici Chuanxiong）, Dahurian angelica root （ Radix Angelicae ）, Dried rehmannia root （ Radix Rehmanniae ）, Scutellaria root （ Radix Scutellariae ）, Licorice root （Radix Glycyrrhizae）

FUNCTIONS

Relieving exterior syndrome, clearing interior heat and alleviating pain.

INDICATION

Syndrome due to the attack of exogenous wind, cold and dampness on the body surface with interior heat, manifested by chill and fever, absence of perspiration, headache with stiff neck, aching pain of the extremities, bitter taste in the mouth with thirst, white and slippery coating of the tongue, floating pulse. It can be used to treat influenza, lumbago, sciatica rheumatic arthritis.

DIRECTIONS

To be taken orally, one pill each time,
twice a day.

PRECAUTION

Spicy and greasy food should be avoided to
take.

047　QINGHAO BIEJIA PIAN （青蒿鳖甲片）

Tablet of Wormwood and Turtle Shell

PRINCIPAL INGREDIENTS

Sweet wormwood (Herba Artemisiae),
Fresh-water turtle shell (Carapax
Trionycis), Dried rehmannia root (Radix
Rehmanniae), Wind-weed rhizome (Rhi-
zoma Anemarrhenae), Tree peony bark
(Cortex Moutan Radicis)

FUNCTIONS

Nourishing Yin and expelling pathogenic
heat from the interior.

INDICATION

Pulmonary tuberculosis and other chronic
consumptive disease related to hyperactivity
of fire due to Yin deficiency manifested with
fever at night and normal in the morning,
absence of perspiration after fever subsides,
polyphagia with emaciation, red tongue

with little coating and rapid pulse.

DIRECTIONS

To be taken orally, 4~6 tablets each time, three times a day.

PRECAUTION

Spicy and greasy food should be avoided to take.

048   CHUANXINLIAN PIAN（穿心莲片）

Andrographis Tablet

PRINCIPAL INGREDIENTS

Andrographis paniculata herb（Herba Andrographitis）

FUNCTIONS

Removing heat and toxic materials and relieving inflammation.

INDICATION

Common cold of wind-head type, tonsillitis, laryngopharyngitis, bronchitis, acute dysentery, acute gastritis, urinary tract infection, pelvic inflammation, otitis media and periodontitis.

DIRECTIONS

To be taken orally, 5 tablets each time, 3~4 times a day.

PRECAUTION

Spicy and greasy food should be avoided to

take.

I -3 Prescriptions for Dispelling Wind
祛风剂

049 XIXIAN WAN （豨莶丸）

Pill of Paulswort

PRINCIPAL INGREDIENTS

Common St. paulswort herb (Herba Siegesbeckiae)

FUNCTIONS

Dispelling wind and removing dampness
from the body, relieving rigidity of muscles
and activating energy flow in the channels
and collaterals.

INDICATION

Arthralgia-syndrome due to pathogenic
wind-cold-dampness, marked by numbness
of the hands and feet, contracture and
spasm of muscles and tendons; stroke manifested as paralysis, hemiplegia and dysphasia, white fur of the tongue, floating and
slow pulse.

DIRECTIONS

To be taken orally, 15～30 pills each time,
twice or three times a day.

PRECAUTION

Spicy and greasy food should be avoided to take.

050　XITONG Pill（豨桐丸）

Pill of Paulswort and Harlequin

PRINCIPAL INGREDIENTS

Common St. paulswort herb (Herba Siegesbeckiae), Harlequin glory bower leaf (Folium Clerodendri Trichotomi)

FUNCTIONS

Expelling wind, dispersing cold and activating the channels and collaterals to relieve pain.

INDICATION

Arthralgia-syndrome due to wind-cold-dampness marked by numb limbs, pantalgia, disability of loins and legs, dysbasia, etc. white fur of the tongue, floating and slow pulse.

DIRECTIONS

To be taken orally, 30 pills each time, twice a day.

PRECAUTION

Spicy and greasy food should be avoided to take.

051　MUGUA WAN（木瓜丸）

Chaenomeles Fruit Pill

PRINCIPAL INGREDIENTS

Chaenomeles Fruit (Fructus Chaenomelis), Chinese angelica root (Radix Angelicae Sinensis), Chuanxiong rhizome (Rhizoma Ligustici Chuanxiong), Dahurian angelica root (Radix Angelicae Dahuricae), Clematis root (Radix Clematidis), Cibot rhizome (Rhizoma Cibotii), Achyranthes root (Radix Achy anthis Bidentatae), Spatholobus stem (Caulis Spatholobi), Ginseng (Radix Ginseng), Sichuan aconite root (Radix Aconiti), Wild Aconite root (Radix Aconiti Kusnezoffii)

FUNCTIONS

Expelling wind, dispersing cold and activating the channels and collaterals to relieve pain.

INDICATION

Arthralgia-syndrome due to wind-cold-dampness marked by numb limbs, pantalgia, disability of loins and legs, dysbasia, etc. pale tongue with white fur, deep and feeble pulse.

DIRECTIONS

To be taken orally, 30 pills each time, twice a day.

The drug is contraindicated for pregnant women.

052 DA HUOLUO WAN （大活络丹）

Large Pill for Activating Channels and Collaterals

PRINCIPAL INGREDIENTS

Ginseng （Radix Ginseng）, Cow-bezoar (Calculus Bovis), Musk (Moschus), Borneol (Borneolum）, Coptis rhizome （Rhizoma Coptidis）, Chinese angelica root （Radix Angelicae Sinensis）, Gastrodia tuber （Rhizoma Gastrodiae）, Scorpion (Scorpio）, Black-tail snake （Zaocys）

FUNCTIONS

Dispelling wind and removing dampness from the body, relieving rigidity muscles and activating energy flow in the channels and collaterals.

INDICATION

Arthralgia-syndrome due to pathogenic wind-cold-dampness, marked by numbness of the hands and feet, contracture and spasm of muscles and tendons; stroke manifested as paralysis, hemiplegia and dysphasia, pale tongue with white fur, deep and feeble pulse.

DIRECTIONS

To be taken orally, one pill each time, twice a day.

PRECAUTION

The pregnant woman is not administrated.

053 GOUPI GAO (狗皮膏)

Dog-Skin Plaster

PRINCIPAL INGREDIENTS

Green tangerine orange peel (Pericarpium Citri Reticulatae Viride), Cloves (Flos Caryophylli), Chuanxiong rhizome (Rhizoma Ligustici Chuanxiong), Chinese angelica root (Radix Angelicae Sinensis), Notopterygium root (Rhizoma seu Radix Notopterygii), Chaulmoogra seed (Semen Chaulmoograe), Pangolin scales (Squama Manitis), Dragon's blood (Resina Draconis), Gastrodia tuber (Rhizoma Gastrodiae), Eucommia bark (Cortex Eucommiae)

FUNCTIONS

Expelling wind and dispersing cold, relaxing muscles and tendons, promoting blood circulation and alleviating pain.

INDICATION

Arthralgia-syndrome due to wind-cold-dampness, pain of loin and lower extremities, numbness of limbs and trunk, traumatic injuries. It can be used to treat rheumatalgia, neuralgia and redness, swelling and pain caused by sprain, etc.

DIRECTIONS

Warm it soft and then apply it to the affected area.

PRECAUTION

It should not be applied to loins and abdomen of women in pregnancy.

054 ZHUIFENG GAO (追风膏)

Rheumatalgia-Relieving Plaster

PRINCIPAL INGREDIENTS

Achyranthes root (Radix Achyranthis Bidentatae), Peach seed (Semen Persicae), Ephedra (Herba Ephedrae), Chinese angelica root (Radix Angelicae Sinensis), Wild aconite root (Radix Aconiti Kusnezoffii), Knoxia root (Radix Knoxiae), Gastrodia tuber (Rhizoma Gastrodiae), Notopterygium root (Rhizome sue Radix Notopterygii), Pangolin scales (Squama Manitis), Asarum herb (Herba Adsari), Lindera root (Radix Linderae)

FUNCTIONS

Expelling wind and dispersing cold, promoting blood circulation to stop pain.

INDICATION

Arthralgia-syndrome due to pathogenic wind-dampness, soreness and pain of back and loins, numbness of limbs. It is used clinically to treat rheumatic arthritis.

DIRECTIONS

Warm it soft and then apply it to the affected area.

PRECAUTION

It should not be applied to loins and abdomen of women in pregnancy.

055 WULI BAHAN SAN （武力拔寒散）

Powder for Expelling Cold with Force

PRINCIPAL INGREDIENTS

Cleome seed (Semen Cleomis), Pericarp of Chinese prickly-ash （ Pericarpium Zanthoxyli）

FUNCTION

Expelling wind and dispersing cold, promoting blood circulation to stop pain.

INDICATION

Arthralgia-syndrome due to pathogenic wind-dampness, soreness andpain of back and loins, numbness of limbs.

DIRECTIONS

To be taken orally, 15g each time, twice a day.

056 XIAOSHUAN ZAIZAO WAN（消栓再造丸）

Restorative Pill for Relieving Thrombus

PRINCIPAL INGREDIENTS

Notoginseng (Radix Notoginseng), Gastrodia tuber (Rhizoma Gastrodiae), Chuanxiong rhizome (Rhizoma Ligustici Chuanxiong)

FUNCTIONS

Nourishing Qi, expelling wind and promoting blood circulation to remove obstruction in the channels and decrease blood lipid.

INDICATION

Apoplexy, hemiplegia, facial hemiparalysis, numbness of limbs. It can be used to treat hemiparalysis and aphasia caused by cerebral embolism, as well as hyperlipidemia.

DIRECTIONS

To be taken orally, one pill each time, twice a day.

PRECAUTION

It should be carefully administrated to the pregnant women.

057 WANGBI CHONGJI （尪痹冲剂）

Infusion for Arthralgia-Syndrome

PRINCIPAL INGREDIENTS

Prepared aconite root （Radix Aconiti Praeparata）,Pubescent angelica root （Radix Angelicae Pubescentis）, Ledebouriella root （Radix Ledebouriellae）, Discos root （Radix Dipsacus）

FUNCTIONS

Dispelling wind-dampness and dredging the channel, arresting pain due to arthralgia-syndrome, tonifying kidney and liver.

INDICATION

Persistent arthralgia-syndrome with deficiency of the liver and kidney marked by cold and pain of loin and knees, limited movement, soreness, weakness or numbness of the joins, pale tongue with white fur and deep and feeble pulse. ,It can be used to deal with chronic arthritis, chronic rheumatic arthritis and rheumatoid arthritis.

DIRECTIONS

To be taken orally after being infused in

boiling water, one packet each time, $2 \sim 3$
times a day.

PRECAUTION

Contraindicated for women in pregnancy.

058　XIAO HUOLUO WAN （小活络丸）

Small Pill for Activating Channels and Collaterals

PRINCIPAL INGREDIENTS

Arisaema with bile （Arisaema cum Bile）,
Prepared Sichuan aconite root （Radix A-
coniti Praeparata ）, Prepared kusnezoff
monkshood root （Radix Aconiti Kusnezoffri
Praeparata）, Earthworm （Lumbricus）, Prepared olibanum （ Resina Olibani Prae-
parata）, Prepared myrrh （Myrrha Praepara-
ta）

FUNCTIONS

Removing pathogenic wind and dampness,
activating energy floe in the channels and
collaterals, treating arthralgia-syndrome.

INDICATION

Artheralgia due to wind-cold- dampness,
pantalgia, numbness andspasm of the
limbs.

DIRECTIONS

To be taken orally with boiled water or yellow rice wine, one pill each time, twice a day.

PRECAUTION

Not advisable for pregnant women.

059 HUOLUO DAN （活络丹）

Pill for Activating Channels and Collaterals

PRINCIPAL INGREDIENTS

Ephedra (Herba Ephedrae), Wild aconite root (Radix Aconiti Kusnezoffii), Pangolin scales (Squama Manitis), Asarum herb (Herba Adsari), Dahurian angelica root (Radix Angelicae Dahuricae), Gypsum (Gypsum Fibrosum), Schizonepeta spike (Spica Schizonepetae), Ligusticum rhizome (Rhizoma Puerariae), White dead silkworm (Bombyx Batryticatus), Gastrodia tuber (Rhizoma Gastrodiae), Arisaema tuber (Rhizoma Arisaematis), Drynaria Rhizome (Rhizoma Drynariae), Agastache herb (Herba Agastachis), Momordica seed (Semen Momordicae), Hematite (Haematitum).

FUNCTIONS

Dispelling wind and removing dampness from the body, relieving rigidity muscles and activating energy flow in the channels and collaterals.

INDICATION

Arthralgia-syndrome due to pathogenic wind-cold-dampness, marked by numbness of the hands and feet, contracture and spasm of muscles and tendons; stroke manifested as paralysis, hemiplegia and dysphasia.

DIRECTIONS

To be taken orally, one pill each time, twice a day.

PRECAUTION

The pregnant woman is not administrated.

060 WUJIAPI JIU （五加皮酒）

Medicated Wine of Acanthopanax

PRINCIPAL INGREDIENTS

Acanthopanax root bark （Cortex Acanthopancis Radicis）, Achyranthes root （Radix Achyranthis Bidentatae）, Chinese angelica root （Radix Angelicae Sinensis）

FUNCTIONS

Expelling pathogenic wind and dredging the channel, dispelling cold and relieving pain.

INDICATION

Arthralgia due to wind-cold-dampness,

numbness of limbs, soreness and pain of muscles and bones, weakness of waist and knees.

DIRECTIONS

To be taken orally, $10 \sim 15$ml each time, three times a day.

PRECAUTION

Not advisable for pregnant women.

061 FENGLIAOXING YAOJIU （冯了性药酒）

Feng Liaoxing Medicated Wine

PRINCIPAL INGREDIENTS

Stem of Erycibe (Caulis Erycibes), Dahurian angelica root (radix Angelicae Dahuricae), Chinese silkvine root bark (Cortex Periplocae Radicis), Ephedra (Herba Ephedrae), Sweet wormwood seed (semen Artemisiae), Chinese angelica root (Radix Angelicae Sinensis), Cinnamon twig (Ramulus Cinnamomi), Common fennel fruit (Fructus Forniculi), Chuanxiong rhizome (Rhizoma Ligustici Chuanxiong), Clematis root (Radix Clematidis), Tetrandra root (Radix Stephaniae Tetrandrae), Capejasmine fruit (Fructus Gardeniae), Notopterygium root (Rhizoma seu Radix Notopterygii), Pubescent angelica root (Radix

Angelicae Pubescentis), White wine

FUNCTIONS

Expelling pathogenic wind and dredging the channel, dispelling cold and relieving pain.

INDICATION

Arthralgia due to wind-cold-dampness, numbness of limbs, soreness and pain of muscles and bones, weakness of waist and knees, recurrence of old trauma.

DIRECTIONS

To be taken orally, 15ml each time, three times a day.

PRECAUTION

Not advisable for pregnant women.

062 GUOGONG JIU (国公酒)

Medicated Wine of Guogong

PRINCIPAL INGREDIENTS

Chinese angelica root (Radix Angelicae Sinensis), Arisaema tuber (Rhizoma Arisaematis), Chaenomeles fruit (Fructus Chaenomelis), Chuanxiong rhizome (Rhizoma Ligustici Chuanxiong), Fragrant solomonseal rhizome (Rhizoma Polygonati Odorati), Notopterygium root (Rhizoma seu Radix Notopterygii)

FUNCTIONS

Expelling pathogenic wind and dampness,
relaxing muscles and tendons and activating
the flow of Qi and blood in the channels and
collaterals.

INDICATION

Arthralgia due to wind-cold-dampness,
numb hands and feet, hemiplegia, facial
paralysis, soreness and pain in the loins and
legs, flaccidity and weakness in the legs,
difficulty in walking.

DIRECTIONS

To be taken orally, 10ml each time, twice a
day.

PRECAUTION

Contraindicated for women in pregnancy.

063 SHANGSHI ZHITONG GAO（伤湿止痛膏）
Adhesive Plaster for Relieving Sprain,
Rheumatalgia and Myalagia

PRINCIPAL INGREDIENTS

Extracted compound liquid for alleviating
pain due to dampness, Methylsalicylate
（Methylsalicylatum）, Menthol （Menth-
olum）, Borneol （Borneolum）, Camphor
(Camphora), Lemongraee extract （Extrac-
tum Herba Cymbopogonis）, Belladonna liquid extract （Extractum Belladonnae Liq-

uidum)

FUNCTIONS

Dispelling wind and dampness and promoting blood circulation to stop pain.

INDICATION

Rheumatic arthritis, myalgia and sprain.

DIRECTIONS

External use, plaster it on the affected area and then change it within 8~12 hours.

PRECAUTION

It should be used with care by pregnant women; not advisable for the patients with adhesive plaster allergy and local ulceration.

064 KANLI SHA （坎离砂）

Sand for Dispelling Wind and Relieving Pain

PRINCIPAL INGREDIENTS

Iron filings, Aconitum root (Radix Aconiti), Chinese angelica root (Radix Angelicae Sinensis), Safflower (Flos Carthami), Achyranthe root (Radix Achyranthis Bidentatae), Ballonflower root (Radix Platycodi), Chaenomeles fruit (Fructus Chaenomelis), Angelica pubescens root (Radix Angelicae Pubescentis)

FUNCTIONS

Dispelling wind and cold, promoting blood circulation to stop pain.

INDICATION

Arthralgia-syndrome due to pathogenic wind-dampness, soreness and pain of back and loins, numbness of limbs and dysbasia. it is used to treat rheumatic arthritis and traumatic injuries.

DIRECTIONS

Warm it and stick it on the affected area.

PRECAUTION

For external use.

065　TIANMA WAN（天麻丸）

Pill of Gastrodia Tuber

PRINCIPAL INGREDIENTS

Gastrodia tuber (Rhizoma Gastrodiae), Notopterygium ('Rhizoma seu Radix Notopterygii), Pubescent angelica root (Radix Angelicae Pubescentis), Eucommia bark (Cortex Eucommiae), Achyranthes root (Radix Achyranthis Bidentatae), Hypoglauca yam (Rhizoma Dioscoreae Hypoglaucae), Prepared aconite root (Radix Aconiti Lateralis Praeparata), Chinese angelica root (Radix Angelicae Sinensis), Rehmannia root

(Radix Rehmanniae), Scrophularia root
(Radix Scrophulariae)

FUNCTIONS

Expelling wind and removing dampness, relaxing muscles and tendons, activating the flow of Qi and blood in the channels and collaterals, promoting blood circulation to relieving pain.

INDICATION

Symptoms due to apoplexy involving the channels such as stiff limbs, numb hands and feet, lassitude and pain in the loins and lags, difficulty in walking; rheumatic arthritis and hemiplegia caused by sequel of stroke.

DIRECTIONS

To be taken orally, one pill each time, twice a day.

PRECAUTION

It should be carefully administrated to the pregnant women.

066 RENSHEN ZAIZAO WAN（人参再造丸）

Restorative Pill of Ginseng

PRINCIPAL INGREDIENTS

Red ginseng (Radix Ginseng), Sandalwood
(Lignum Santali), Prepared rehmannia root

(Radix Rehmanniae Praeparata), Amber
(Succinum), Gastrodia tuber (Rhizoma
Gastrodiae), Chinese angelica root (Radix
Angelicae Sinensis), Clematis root (Radix
Clematidis), Long-noded pit viper (Agk-
istrodon), Tortoris plastron (Plastrum Tes-
tudinis), Batryticated silkworm (Bombyx
Batrydicatus), Dragon's blood (Resina Dra-
conis), Cow-bezoar (Calculus Bovis), Musk
(Moschus), Borneol (Borneolum),
Tabasheer (Concretio Silices Bambusae)

FUNCTIONS

Nourishing Qi, promoting blood circulation
to remove stasis, dispelling pathogenic wind
and removing obstruction in the channels.

INDICATION

Apoplexy, hemiplegia, facial hemiparalysis, numbness of limbs, pain in loins and
knees. It has significant effect on hemiparalysis and aphasia caused by cerebral embolism.

DIRECTIONS

To be taken orally, one pill each time,
twice a day.

PRECAUTION

Not advised for pregnant woman.

067 HUITIAN ZAIZAO WAN （回天再造丸）

Restorative Pill with Tremendous Power

PRINCIPAL INGREDIENTS

Ginseng （Radix Ginseng）, Cow-bezoar (Calculus Bovis), Musk (Moschus), Gastrodia tuber (Rhizoma Gastrodiae）, Dragon's blood (Resina Draconis）, Goral Blood (Sanguis Naemorhedi)

FUNCTIONS

Dispelling wind, resolving phlegm and promoting blood circulation to remove obstruction in the channels.

INDICATION

Hemiplegia, facial hemiparalysis, soreness in loins and legs, numbness of limbs.

DIRECTIONS

To be taken orally, one pill each time, twice a day.

PRECAUTION

Spicy and greasy food should be avoided to take.

068 XIXIAN FENGSHI WAN （豨莶风湿丸）

Pill of Paulswort for Expelling Wind-Cold

PRINCIPAL INGREDIENTS

Common St. paulswort herb (Herba Siegesbeckiae）, Loranthus mulberry mistletoe

(Ramulus Loranthis), Tetrandra root
(Radix Stephaniae Tetrandrae), Clematis
root (Radix Clematidis), Pagodatree twig
(Ramulus Sophorae), Mulberry twig (Ramulus Mori)

FUNCTIONS

Dispelling wind and removing dampness,
relieving, pain due to arthralgia-syndrome,
tonifying the liver and kidney.

INDICATION

Arthralgia-syndrome due to pathogenic
wind-cold-dampness, marked by numbness,
cold and pain of the hands and feet, contracture and spasm of muscles and tendons,
limited movement, soreness weakness of
the joins, white fur of the tongue, deep,
slow and feeble pulse.

DIRECTIONS

To be taken orally, Adults one pill each
time, twice a day; Children above 7 years
old taken 1/2 dosage of the adult; lower 7
years old taken 1/3 dosage of the adult.

PRECAUTION

The pregnant woman is not administrated.

069　TUSU JIU （屠苏酒）

Medicated Wine of Tusu

PRINCIPAL INGREDIENTS

Cinnamon bark (Cortex Cinnamoni), Lede-douriella root (Radix Ledebouriellae), Hypoglauca yam (Rhizoma Dioscoreae Hypoglaucae), Platycodon root (Radix Platycodi), Rhubarb (Radix et Rhizoma Rhei), Sappan wood (Lignum Sappan), Pericarp of Chinese prickly-ash (Pericarpium Zanthoxyli), Aconitum root (Radix Aconiti)

FUNCTIONS

Expelling pathogenic wind and cold.

INDICATION

Arthralgia due to wind-cold-dampness, contracture and spasm of tendons, numbness of hands and feet, pain in the shoulder and back, lumbago, cold legs, hemiplegia, soreness and pain in joints. Also used to treat exterior syndrome due to exopathic wind- cold marked by chill, fever, headache.

DIRECTIONS

To be taken orally, 10ml each time, twice a day.

PRECAUTION

Contraindicated for women in pregnant.

070 SHEDAN ZHUIFENG WAN（蛇胆追风丸）

Pill of Snake Bile for Expelling Wind

PRINCIPAL INGREDIENTS

Snake bile (Bilis Serpentis), Earthworm (Lumbricus), Pubescent angelica root (Radix Angelicae Pubescentis), Chinese angelica root (Radix Angelicae Sinensis), Arisaema with bile (Arisaema cum Bile), Prepared Sichuan aconite root (Radix Aconiti Praeparata), Prepared kusnezoff monkshood (Radix Aconiti Kusnezoffi Praeparata), Ledebouriella root (Radix Ledebouriellae), Chuanxiong rhizome (Rhizoma Ligustici Chuanxiong), Pinellia tuber (Rhizoma Pinelliae)

FUNCTIONS

Expelling wind and eliminating phlegm, activating energy flow in the channels and collaterals.

INDICATION

Arthralgia due to wind-cold-dampness and blood stasis marked by contracture and spasm of tendons, numbness of hands and feet, pain in the shoulder and back, lumbago, cold and weak legs, hemiplegia, soreness and pain in joints.

DIRECTIONS

To be taken orally, 8～10 pills each time,

twice a day.

PRECAUTION

Spicy and greasy food should be avoided to take.

071 TIANMA TOUTENG PIAN (天麻头痛片)

Tablet of Gastrodia Tuber for Headache

PRINCIPAL INGREDIENTS

Gastrodia tuber (Rhizoma Gastrodiae), Chinese angelica root (Radix Angelicae Sinensis), Chuanxiong rhizome (Rhizoma Ligustici Chuanxiong), Root of angelica dahurica (Radix Angelicae Dahuricae), Frankincense (Resina Olibani)

FUNCTIONS

Expelling wind and promoting blood circulation to relieving pain.

INDICATION

Headaches of traumatic injury and internal diseases caused by wind and blood stasis.

DIRECTIONS

To be taken orally, 4~6 tablets each time, twice a day.

PRECAUTION

It should be carefully administrated to the pregnant women.

072 QISHE YAOJIU (蕲蛇药酒)

Medicated Wine of Agkistrodon

PRINCIPAL INGREDIENTS

Agkistrodon (Agkistrodon), Lededouriella root (Radix Ledebouriellae), Chinese angelica root (Radix Angelicae Sinensis), Notopterygium root (Rhizoma seu Radix Notopterygii), Large-leaf gentian root (Radix Gentianae Macrophyllae), Acanthopancis root bark (Cortex Acanthopancis), Gastrodia tuber (Rhizoma Gastrodiae), Carthamus flower (Flos Carthami)

FUNCTIONS

Expelling pathogenic wind and cold, promoting blood circulating to remove stasis.

INDICATION

Arthralgia due to wind-cold-dampness and blood stasis marked by contracture and spasm of tendons, numbness of hands and feet, pain in the shoulder and back, lumbago, cold legs, hemiplegia, soreness and pain in joints.

DIRECTIONS

To be taken orally, 10ml each time, twice a day.

PRECAUTION

Contraindicated for women in pregnant.

073　KANGSHUAN ZAIZAO WAN （抗栓再造丸）

Restorative Pill for Anti-Thrombus

PRINCIPAL INGREDIENTS

Red ginseng (Radix Ginseng Rubra), Astragalus root (Radix Astragali seu Hedysari), Cow-bezoar (Calculus Bovis), Musk (Moschus), Borneol (Borneolum)

FUNCTIONS

Promoting blood circulation to remove blood stasis, dispelling pathogenic wind and relieving pain and spasm.

INDICATION

Apoplexy, hemiplegia, facial hemiparalysis, limb pain and spasm.

DIRECTIONS

To be taken orally, one pill each time, twice a day.

PRECAUTION

Not advised for pregnant women.

74　XIAOSHUAN TONGLUO PIAN （消栓通络片）

Tablet for Dissolving Thrombus and Clearing Channel

PRINCIPAL INGREDIENTS

Notoginseng (Radix Notoginseng), Astragalus root (Radix Astragali), Curcuma root (Radix Curcumae), Cassia twig (Ramulus Cinnamomi)

FUNCTIONS

Expelling wind and promoting blood circulation to relieving pain.

INDICATION

Headaches of traumatic injury and internal diseases caused by wind and blood stasis.

DIRECTIONS

To be taken orally, 4~6 tablets each time, twice a day.

PRECAUTION

It should be carefully administrated to the pregnant women.

075 HUATUO ZAIZAO WAN （华佗再造丸）

Huatuo Restorative Pill

PRINCIPAL INGREDIENTS

Red ginseng (Radix Ginseng Rubra), Chinese angelica root (Radix Angelicae Sinensis),Chuanxiong rhizome (Rhizoma Ligustici Chuanxiong),Safflower (Flos Carthami), Chinese magnoliavine fruit (Fructus Schisandrae), Strychnos seed (Semen Strychni), Borneol (Borneolum), Arusaema tuber (Rhizoma Gastrodiae)

FUNCTIONS

Promoting blood circulation to remove stasis, Removing dampness and obstruction in the channels, dispelling pathogenic wind and relieving pain.

INDICATION

Hemiplegia of acute and sequelae of apoplexy, deviation of eye and mouth, intricate and obscure speech, involuntary drooling, atrophy and disability of limbs, deep-red or light purple tongue and taut pulse.

DIRECTIONS

To be taken orally, 8g each time, 2 ~ 3 times a day.

PRECAUTION

Not advised for pregnant women. Spicy and greasy food should be avoided to take.

I-4 Prescriptions for Eliminating Wetness
祛湿剂

076 LIUYI SAN（六一散）

Six to One Powder

PRINCIPAL INGREDIENTS

Talc (Talcum), Licorice root (Radix Glycyrrhizae)

FUNCTION

Clearing away summer-heat and eliminating wetness

INDICATIONS

Syndrome of wetness in the summer, syndrome of heat and wetness, and Lin syndrome (stranguria) due to heat and wetness retained in the lower JIAO, manifested as fever, sweating, thirst, vexation, oliguria with deep color, red tongue with yellow coating, rapid and slippery pulse; miliaria and eczema caused by heat and wetness.

DIRECTIONS

To be taken orally for clearing away heat in summer, heat and wetness, 6 ~ 9g each time, twice a day. For miliaria and eczema, to be used externally.

PRECAUTION

As it is cold in nature, it should be carefully administered to patient with cold constitution.

077 YIYUAN SAN（益元散）

Powder for Restoring Health

PRINCIPAL INGREDIENTS

Talc (Talcum), Licorice root (Radix Glycyrrhizae)

FUNCTIONS

Clearing away summer-heat, eliminating wetness, easing anxiety, calming fright, tranquilizing the mind.

INDICATIONS

Syndrome of summer-heat and wetness with irritability, markedly fever, sweating, lassitude, thirst, vomiting, diarrhea, oliguria with deep color, red tongue with yellow coating, rapid and slippery pulse as well as palpitation and irritability.

DIRECTIONS

To be taken orally, 6g each time, 1～2 times a day.

PRECAUTION

Avoid raw, cool and greasy food.

078   DAYUAN WAN（达原丸）

Deep Reaching Pill

PRINCIPAL INGREDIENTS

Betel nut (Semen Arecae), Bark of official magnolia （Cortex Magnoliae Officinalis）, Caoguo （Fructus Tsaoko）, Rhizome of wind-weed (Rhizoma Anemarrhenae), Root of herbaceous peony(Radix Paeoniae Alba), Skullcap (Radix Scutellariae), Licorice root

(Radix Glycyrrhizae)

FUNCTIONS

Removing turbid pathogenic factor, clearing away heat and detoxicating.

INDICATION

A lternate attacks of chill and fever, accompanying with headache, irritability, fullness and oppression in the chest, nausea, fullness and distention in the abdomen, viscid stool with terribly foul odor, deep and red tongue with thick and greasy coating, wiry and rapid pulse due to influenza, malaria and typhoid fever, in traditional Chinese medicine differentiation belong to wet and warm syndrome.

DIRECTIONS

To be taken orally, one pill each time, twice a day.

PRECAUTION

Spicy and greasy food should be avoided to take.

079　ERMIAO WAN（二妙丸）

Pill of Two Wonderful Drugs

PRINCIPAL INGREDIENTS

Chinese atractylodes（Rhizoma Atractylodis）, Corktree（Cortex Phellodendri）

FUNCTIONS

Clearing away heat and wetness from lower JIAO.

INDICATIONS

Fullness and oppression in the chest, poor appetite, fullness and distention in the abdomen, heavy limbs, or lassitude, deep colored urine, yellow and greasy tongue coating, soft and rapid pulse caused by heat and wetness retained in the lower JIAO. Rheumatic fever, rheumatic arthritis, polyneuritis show above symptoms.

DIRECTIONS

To be taken orally, 6~9g each time, three times a day.

PRECAUTION

Greasy and fried food should be avoided to take, it is not advisable for the patient whose constitution is belonged to YIN deficiency.

080 SANMIAO WAN (三妙丸)

Pill of Three Wonderful Drugs

PRINCIPAL INGREDIENTS

Chinese atractylodes (Rhizoma Atractylodis), Corktree (Cortex Phellodendri), Bidentate achyranthes (Radix Achyranthis

Bidentatae)

FUNCTIONS

Clearing away heat and wetness from lower JIAO.

INDICATIONS

BI syndrome due to wetness and heat, manifested as swelling pain with erythema in the knee and angle, and accompanying with lassitude, poor appetite, yellow and greasy tongue coating, soft and slippery pulse; eczema and itch in the lower limbs, and beriberi with swelling pain; leukorrhea caused by heat and wetness retained in the lower JIAO, manifested as yellow leukorrhea with foul odor, itch in the pudendum, soreness and weakness in the loins and knees, oliguria with deep color, bitter mouth, dry throat, white and greasy, or yellow and greasy tonguecoating, slippery and rapid pulse.

DIRECTIONS

To be taken orally, 9g each time, twice a day. For the child who is over7 years old, it should be taken the half of dosage, for who is between three to seven, one third of dosage can be taken.

PRECAUTION

It is contraindicated in women with menorrhagia, or pregnant women.

081 BIXIE FENQING WAN (萆薢分清丸)

Separating Pill with Yam.

PRINCIPAL INGREDIENTS

Yam (Rhizoma Dioscoreae), Galangal fruit
(Fructus Alpiniae Oxyphyllae), Root of
three-nerved spicebush (Radix Linderae),
Grass-leaved sweetflag (Rhizoma Acori
Graminei), Tuckahoe (Poria), Licorice root
(Radix Glycyrrhizae)

FUNCTIONS

Warming the kidney to promote diuresis,
separating the nutrition and the waste, e-
liminating wetness.

INDICATIONS

Frequent urination with cloudy rice-water
like or oily urine, accompanying with dizzy,
weakness, lassitude, soreness and soft of
knee and waist, pale complexion, cold
limbs, pale tongue with greasy coating,
deep and thready, or weak pulse due to deficiency of kidney-YANG and retention of
wetness in the body. Chronic prostatitis and
chyluria show above symptoms.

DIRECTIONS

To be taken orally, 6g each time, twice a day. For the child who is over 7 years old, it should be taken the half of dosage, for who is between three to seven, one third of dosage can be taken.

PRECAUTION

Raw and cool food should be avoided to taken.

082　BUHUANJIN ZHENGQI SAN（不换金正气散）

Wonderful Powder for Restoring Health

PRINCIPAL INGREDIENTS

Dried old orange peel （Pericarpium Citri Reticulatae）, Pinellia （Rhizoma Pinelliae）, Bark of official magnolia （Cortex Magnoliae Officianlis）, Chinese atractylodes （Rhizoma Atractylodis）, Wrinkled gianthyssop （Herba Agastachis）, Licorice root （Radix Glycyrrhizae）

FUNCTIONS

Eliminating wetness and invigorating the spleen.

INDICATIONS

Retention of wetness in the spleen and stomach, manifested by stuffiness, and distention in the abdomen,, eructation,, acid

regurgitation, vomiting, diarrhea, or tastelessness, poor appetite, heaviness sensation
in the limbs, enlargement tongue with teeth
marks, and thick, white and greasy coating, slow pulse. Dyspepsia, gastrointestinal dysfunction, chronic gastritis show
above symptoms.

DIRECTIONS

To be taken orally, 6~9g each time, three
times a day.

PRECAUTION

Raw, cool and greasy food should be avoided to take.

083   LIUHE DINGZHONG WAN (六合定中丸)

Pill for Easing the Middle JIAO

PRINCIPAL INGREDIENTS

Wrinkled gianthyssop (Herba Agastachis),
Leaf of purple perilla (Folium Perillae),
Tuckahoe (Poria), Bean of white hyacinth
dolichos (Semen Dolichoris Album), Dried
old orange peel (Pericarpium Citri Reticulatae), Bark of official magnolia (Cortex
Magnoliae Officinalis), Chinese flowering
quince (Fructus Chaenomelis), Fruit of citron or trifoliate orange (Fructus Aurantii),

Sandal wood (Lignum Santali), Malt (Fructus Hordei Germinatus), Rice-grain sprout (Fructus Oryzae Germinatus), Fruit of hawthorn (Fructus Crataegi), Costusroot (Radix Saussureae Lappae), Herb huichow elsholtzia (Herba Elscholtziaeseu Moslae), Medicated leaven (Massa Medicata Fermentata), Root of ballonflower (Radix Platycodi), Licorice root (Radix Glycyrrhizae)

FUNCTIONS

Clearing away summer-heat to relieve exterior syndrome, regulating the middle JIAO to arrest vomiting, invigorating the spleen to stop diarrhea.

INDICATIONS

Disease caused by heat and wetness in the summer, improper diet, taking raw and cool food, caused retention of food and fluid in the stomach, manifested as vomiting, diarrhea, nausea, pain in the abdomen with distention and stuffiness, and refusing to press, cold limbs, white and greasy tongue coating, soft and slippery pulse, or floating pulse. Acute gastritis and acute gastroenteritis show above symptoms.

DIRECTIONS

To be taken orally, one pill each time, three times a day.

PRECAUTION

Raw, cool, oily and greasy food should be avoided to take, and it is contraindicated in pregnant women.

084 WULING WAN (五苓丸)

Five Drug Pill with Poria

PRINCIPAL INGREDIENTS

Bark of Chinese cassia tree (Cortex Cinnamomi), Large-headed atractylodes (Rhizoma Atractylodis Macrocephalae), Oriental water plantain (Rhizoma Alismatis), Tuckahoe (Poria), Umbellate pore fungus (Polyporus Umbellatus)

FUNCTIONS

Warming YANG and invigorating the spleen to promote diuresis and eliminate wetness.

INDICATIONS

Deficiency of Yang and retention of water in the body, marked by edema, oliguria, or diarrhea with oliguria, aversion to cold, or borborygmus, soreness of waist, pale tongue with white coating. Chronic nephritis show above symptoms.

DIRECTIONS

To be taken orally, 6g each time, twice a day. For the child who is over 7 years old, it should be taken the half of dosage, for who is between three to seven, one third of dosage can be taken.

PRECAUTION

The recipe is contraindicated in patients with difficulty of urination due to deficiency of YIN, and edema caused by heat.

085 BANXIA TIANMA WAN (半夏天麻丸)

Pill with Pinellia and Gastrodia

PRINCIPAL INGREDIENTS

Pinellia (Rhizoma Pinelliae), Tuber of elevated gastrodia (Rhizoma Gastrodiae), Large-headed atractylodes (Rhizoma Atractylodis macrocephalae), Milk veteh (Radix Astragali seu Hedysari), Ginseng (Radix Ginseng), Tuckahoe (Poria), Oriental water plantain (Rhizoma Alismatis), Chinese atractylodes (Rhizoma Atractylodis), Corktree (Cortex Phellodendri), Medicated leaven(Massa Medicata Fermentata), Dried old orange peel (Pericarpium Citri Reticulatae), Malt (Fructus Hordei Germinatus)

FUNCTIONS

Invigorating the spleen to eliminate wetness and expel phlegm and calming the endogenous wind.

INDICATIONS

Headache, dizziness, oppression and distention in the chest, nausea, vomiting with phlegm and saliva, weakness, lassitude, loose stool, thick and greasy tongue coating, wiry and slippery pulse caused by phlegm.

DIRECTIONS

To be taken orally, 6g each time, twice a day.

PRECAUTION

It should be avoided to take while dizziness and headache are caused by hyperactivity of the liver-YANG.

086 XIAO WENZHONG WAN （小温中丸）

Minor Pill for Warming the Middle JIAO

PRINCIPAL INGREDIENTS

Tuckahoe (Poria), Pinellia (Rhizoma Pinelliae), Dried old orange peel (Pericarpium Citri Reticulatae), Medicated leaven (Massa Medicata Fermentata), Chinese goldthread (Rhizoma Coptidis), Large-headed atractylodes (Rhizoma Atractylodis Macrocep-ha-lae), Nutgrass flatsedge (Rhizoma Cyperi), Licorice root (Radix Glycyrrhizae), Sand of iron (Fe), Flavescent sophora root (Radix Sophorae Flavescentis)

FUNCTIONS

Invigorating the spleen to relieving the edema, and clearing away heat and eliminating wetness.

INDICATIONS

Sallow complexion, lassitude, weakness, abdominal distention and stuffiness, poor appetite, dried mouth, but not willing to drink water, edema in the lower limbs, deep colored urine, viscose stool, yellow and greasy tongue coating, slippery and rapid pulse caused by deficiency of the spleen with wetness and heat.

DIRECTIONS

To be taken orally, 6g each time, three times a day. For the child who is over 7 years old, it should be taken the half of dosage.

PRECAUTION

Never is it administered for pregnant women, moreover, it is better to take the food with few salt.

087 XIANGSHA PINGWEI CHONGJI（香砂平胃冲剂）

Infusion with Nutgrass Flatsedge and Amomun Fruit for Easing the Stomach

PRINCIPAL INGREDIENTS

Dried old orange peel（Pericarpium Citri Reticulatae）, Chinese atractylodes（Rhizoma Atractylodis）, Bark of official magnolia（Cortex Magnoliae Officinalis）, Nutgrass flatsedge（Rhizoma Cyperi）, Amomun fruit（Fructus Amomi）, Licorice root（Radix Glycyrrhizae）

FUNCTIONS

Depriving wetness, invigorating the spleen, promoting Qi circulation, regulating the stomach, warming middle JIAO, and relieving pain.

INDICATIONS

Distention and fullness in the stomach, or accompanying with pain, nausea, vomiting, poor appetite, eructation, acid regurgitation, diarrhea, tastelessness, white, thick and greasy tongue coating, and soft and floating pulse, or accompanying with heavy limbs, lassitude, drowsiness due to impairment of the spleen, food and wetness retention caused by improper diet.

DIRECTIONS

To be taken orally, one pack (10g) each time, three times a day.

PRECAUTION

It is forbidden to take raw, cold, oily, greasy and fried food.

088 SHENYAN XIAOZHONG PIAN （肾炎消肿片）

Tablet for Detumescence in Nephritis

PRINCIPAL INGREDIENTS

Chinese atractylodes (Rhizoma Atractylodis). Dried old orange peel (Pericarpium Citri Reticulatae). Wujiapi (Cortex Acanthopanacis Radicis). Tuckaohe (Poria). Ginger peel (Exocarpium Zingiberis Recens). Shell of areca nut (Pericarpium Arecae). Water melon (Exocarpium Citrulli). Oriental water plantain (Rhizoma Alismatis). Corktree (Cortex Phellodendri). Seed of peppertree pricklyash (Semen Zanthoxyli). Motherwort (Herba Leonuri)

FUNCTIONS

Invigorating the spleen, eliminating wetness, warming YANG and diuresis.

INDICATIONS

Nephritis, whose differentiation is wetness retention in the spleen, manifested as edema in the limbs, facial edema in the morning, heavy limbs, oliguria, stuffiness and distension in the abdomen, poor appetite, white and greasy tongue coating, and deep and slow pulse.

DIRECTIONS

To be taken orally, 5 tablets each time, three times a day, and take 20 days as a course, treatment needs three courses.

PRECAUTION

It is contraindicated in patient who is deficient.

I-5 Prescriptions for Promoting Digestion
消导剂

089 XIANGSHA YANGWEI WAN (香砂养胃丸)

Pill of Nutgrass Flatsedge and Amomum Fruit for Well-Preserving the Stomach.

PRINCIPAL INGREDIENTS

Nutgrass flatsedge (Rhizoma Cyperi), Amomum fruit (Fructus Amomi), Large-headed atractylodes (Rhizoma Atractylodis Macrocephalae), Dried old orange peel (Pericarpium Citri Reticulatae), Wrinkled gianthyssop (Herba Agastachis), Tuckahoe (Poria), Katsumadai seed (Semen Álpiniae Katsumadai), Bark of official magnolia (Cortex Magnoliae Officinalis), Fruit of immature bitter orange (Fructus Aurantii Immaturus), Pinellia (Rhizoma Pinelliae), Costusroot (Radix Saussureae Lappae), Licorice root (Radix Glycyrrhizae)

FUNCTIONS

Invigorating the spleen, regulating the spleen and stomach, eliminating wetness with fragrant drugs, relieving the distension of abdomen.

INDICATIONS

Distention and fullness in the chest and abdomen, stomachache, diarrhea, vomiting, dyspepsia, sallow complexion, lassitude, weakness, shortness of breath, disinclination to talk, eructation, vomiting, borborygmus, pale tongue with white and greasy coating, deep and slow pulse caused by deficiency of Qi, retardation of wetness and stagnation of Qi.

DIRECTIONS

To be taken orally, 6g each time, three times a day.

PRECAUTION

It should be avoided to take the cold and raw food, and to be angry during the treatment.

090   MUXIANG SHUNQi WAN (木香顺气丸)

Pill with Costusroot for Smoothing Qi

PRINCIPAL INGREDIENTS

Costusroot (Radix Saussureae Lappae), Bark of official magnolia (Cortex Magnoliae Officinalis), Amomum fruit (Fructus Amomi), Fruit of bitter orange (Fructus Aurantii), Nutgrass flatsedge (Rhizoma Cyperi), Chinese atractylodes (Rhizoma Atractylodis), Dried old orange peel (Pericarpium Citri Reticulatae), Dried green orange peel (Pericarpium Citri Reticulatae Viride), Betel nut (Semen Arecae), Licorice root (Radix Glycyrrhizae), Ginger (Rhizoma Zingiberis Recens)

FUNCTIONS

Smoothing Qi and promoting Qi circulation, depriving the wetness and invigorating the spleen.

INDICATIONS

Fullness and oppression in the chest and abdomen, abdominal pain and distension, nausea, vomiting, poor appetite, eructation, acid regurgitation, constipation, red tongue with thick, white and greasy coating, deep and slippery pulse due to the stagnation of Qi and dyspepsia.

DIRECTIONS

To be taken orally, 6~9g each time, 2~3 times a day.

PRECAUTION

It should be avoided to take, for who has the stagnation of Qi with heat and the deficiency of YIN, since this formula is full of fragrant drugs. Raw, cold and greasy food should be avoided to take. And it is contraindicated in pregnant women.

091　DA SHANZHA WAN（大山楂丸）

Bigger Pill with Hawthron

PRINCIPAL INGREDIENTS

Fruit of hawthorn (Fructus Crataegi), Malt (Fructus Hordei Germinatus), Medicated leaven (Massa Medicata Fermentata), Granulated sugar (Sacharum)

FUNCTIONS

Increasing appetite and promoting digestion.

INDICATIONS

Dyspepsia, distension and oppression in the abdomen. Coronary heart disease, hyperlipemia and deficiency of vitamin B shows above symptoms.

DIRECTIONS

To be taken orally, 1~2 pills each time, three times a day.

PRECAUTION

Greasy food should be avoided to take, and it is contraindicated in hyperhydrochloria.

092 ZHISHI DAOZHI WAN（枳实导滞丸）

Pill of Immature Bitter Orange for Removing Stagnancy

PRINCIPAL INGREDIENTS

Fruit of immature bitter orange (Fructus Aurantii Immaturus), Rhubarb (Radix et Rhizoma Rhei), Chinese goldthread (Rhizoma Coptidis), Skullcap (Radix Scutellariae), Tuckahoe (Poria), Oriental water plantain (Rhizoma Alismatis), Medicated leaven (Massa Medicata Fermentata), Large-headed atractylodes (Rhizoma Atractylodis Macrocephalae)

FUNCTIONS

Promoting digestion to remove stagnated food and eliminating wetness and heat.

INDICATIONS

Syndrome due to the stagnation of food and wetness and heat retained manifested as fullness, and oppression in the, chest, and abdomen, abdominal pain, dysentery, diarrhea, tenesmus, or constipation, oliguria with deep color, red tongue with yellow and greasy coating, slippery and rapid pulse.

DIRECTIONS

To be taken orally, 9g each time, twice a day.

PRECAUTION

Raw, cold and greasy food should be avoided to take.

093   WUBEI SAN（乌贝散）

Powder of Fritillary Bulb and Cuttlebone

PRINCIPAL INGREDIENTS

Fritillary bulb （Bulbus Fritillariae Thunbergii）, Cuttlebone （ Os Sepiellae seu Sepiae）

FUNCTIONS

Clearing away heat, expelling phlegm, and reducing acid to relieve pain.

INDICATIONS

Syndrome of phlegm and heat retained, in middle JIAO, and abnormal rising of stomach Qi manifested as stomachache concerned with diet, or pain after meals, or while hunger, which may be relieved after meals, acid regurgitation, yellow tongue coating, slippery and rapid pulse.

DIRECTIONS

To be taken orally, 2～3g each time, 2～3 times a day.

PRECAUTION

Eating and drinking should be moderated, spicy and greasy should be avoided to take, and monkshood is forbidden to be taken during taking this powder.

094　BAO HE WAN （保和丸）

Lenitive Pill

PRINCIPAL INGREDIENTS

Fruit of hawthorn (Fructus Crataegi), Medicated leaven （Massa Medicata Fermentata）, Chinese radish seed （Semen Raphani）, Malt (Fructus Hordei Germinatus), Pinellia (Rhizoma Pinelliae), Dried old orange peel （Pericarpium Citri Reticulatae）, Tuckahoe (Poria), Weeping forsythia (Fructus Forsythiae)

FUNCTIONS

Promoting digestion and regulating the

stomach and spleen.

INDICATIONS

Distension and fullness in the abdomen, eructation with fetid odor, acid regurgitation, nausea, vomiting, loss of appetite, or diarrhea, dysentery caused by retention of food, thick and greasy tongue coating, slippery pulse due to dyspepsia.

DIRECTIONS

To be taken orally, 6g each time, twice a day.

PRECAUTION

It should be avoided to take for the deficiency of spleen without retention of food.

095   JIAWEI BAOHE WAN (加味保和丸)

Modified Lenitive Pill

PRINCIPAL INGREDIENTS

Tuckahoe (Poria), Fruit of hawthorn (Fructus Crataegi), Large-headed atractylodes (Rhizoma Atractylodis Macrocephalae), Medicated leaven (Massa Medicata Fermentata), Dried old orange peel (Pericarpium Citri Reticulatae), Pinellia (Rhizoma Pinelliae), Bark of official magnolia (Cortex Magnoliae Officinalis), Malt (Fructus Hordei Germinatus), Nutgrass flatsedge

(Rhizoma Cyperi), Fruit of immature bitter orange (Fructus Aurantii Immaturus), Fruit of citron or tifoliate orange (Fructus Aurantii)

FUNCTIONS

Promoting digestion, removing stagnancy, invigorating the spleen and eliminating wetness.

INDICATIONS

Stomachache, abdominal pain, stuffiness and fullness in the chest, eructation with fetid odor, loss of appetite, nausea, acid regurgitation, retention of food, diarrhea, thick, white and greasy tongue coating, slippery pulse.

DIRECTIONS

To be take orally, 6～12 each time, three times a day.

PRECAUTION

Indigestible food such as oily, greasy, sticky foods and etc. should be avoided to take.

096 YUEJU BAOHE WAN （越鞠保和丸）

Lenitive Pill for Relieving Stagnancy

PRINCIPAL INGREDIENTS

Nutgrass flatsedge (Rhizoma Cyperi),Capejasmine (Fructus Gardeniae), Chinese atractylodes (Rhizoma Atractylodis), Chuanxiong (Rhizoma Ligustici Chuanxiong), Costusroot (Radix Saussureae Lappae), Medicated leaven (Massa Medicata Fermentata), Betel nut (Semen Arecae)

FUNCTIONS

Promoting Qi circulation to disperse the depressed Qi, invigorating the spleen to promote digestion.

INDICATIONS

Syndromes of Qi stagnation and food retention manifested as distension and pain in the chest and hypochondrium, stuffiness and fullness in the abdomen, retention of food, eructation with fetid odor, gastric discomfort with acid regurgitation, loss of appetite, nausea, thick and greasy tongue coating, wiry and slippery pulse.

DIRECTIONS

To be taken orally, 6g each time, twice a day.

PRECAUTION

It is contraindicated in pregnant women.

097 QIPI WAN （启脾丸）

Pill for Activating the Spleen

PRINCIPAL INGREDIENTS

Large-heated atractylodes (Rhizoma A-tractylodis Macrocephalae), Ginseng (Radix Ginseng), Tuckahoe (Poria), Dried old orange peel (Pericarpium Citri Reticulatae), Licorice root (Radix Glycyrrhizae), Chinese yam rhizome (Rhizoma Dioscoreae), Fruit of hawthorn (Fructus Crataegi), Malt (Fructus Hordei Germinatus), Oriental water plantain (Rhizoma Alismatis), Medicated leaven (Massa Medicata Fermentata), Hindu lotus seed (Semen Nelumbinis)

FUNCTIONS

Invigorating the spleen, regulating the stomach, promoting digestion and stopping diarrhea.

INDICATIONS

Syndromes of the spleen deficiency and food retention manifested as stuffiness, distension and pain in the chest and abdomen, loss of appetite, nausea, vomiting, eructation with fetid odor,, acid regurgitation, loose stool with foul smell, and accompanying with lassitude, sallow complexion, pale tongue with white, thick and greasy coating, weak and slow pulse.

DIRECTIONS

To be taken orally, one pill each time, 2～3
times a day.

PRECAUTION

Cold, raw and greasy food should be avoided to take.

098   ZISHENG WAN （资生丸）

Supplying Pill

PRINCIPAL INGREDIENTS

Hindu lotus seed (Semen Nelumbinis), Chi-
nese yam rhizome (Rhizoma Dioscoreae),
Fruit of hawthorn (Fructus Crataegi),
Tuckahoe (Poria), Dangshen (Radix
Codonopsis Pilosulae), Large-headed a-
tractylodes (Rhizoma Atractylodis Macro-
cephalae), Gordon euryale (Semen
Euryales), Job's tears (Semen Coicis),
Wrinklws gianthyssop (Herba Agastachis),
Bean of white hyacinth dolichos (Semen
Dolichoris Album), Root of balloon flower
(Radix Platycodi), Medicated leaven (Mas-
sa Medicata Fermentata), Galangal fruit
(Fructus Galangae), Chinese goldthread
(Rhizoma Coptidis), Malt (Fructus Hordei
Germinatus)

FUNCTIONS

Invigorating the spleen to resolve wetness,

promoting digestion to stop diarrhea.

INDICATIONS

Fullness and stuffiness in the chest and abdomen, gastric discomfort, poor appetite, nausea, vomiting, loose stool, sallow complexion, lassitude, weakness, greasy and yellowish tongue coating, deep, thready and weak pulse, or slow pulse caused by deficiency of spleen accompanying with wetness and heat retained.

DIRECTIONS

To be taken orally, 3g each time, three times a day.

PRECAUTION

Raw, cold and greasy food should be avoided to take during taking this medicine.

099　MUXIANG BINLANG WAN（木香槟榔丸）

Pill with Costusroot and Betel Nut

PRINCIPAL INGREDIENTS

Costusroot (Radix Saussureae Lappae), Betel nut (Semen Arecae), Fruit of citron or trifoliate orange (Fructus Aurantii), Dried old orange peel (Pericarpium Citri Reticulatae), Dried green orange peel (Pericarpium Citri Reticulatae Viride), Nutgrass foatsedge (Rhizoma Cyperi), Burreed (Rhizoma Sparganii), Zedoary turmeric (Rhizoma Zedoariae), Chinese goldthread (Rhizoma Coptidis), Corktree (Cortex Phellodendri), Rhubarb (Radix et Rhizoma Rhei), Mirabilite (Mirabilitum), Morning glory seed (Semen Pharbitidis)

FUNCTIONS

Promoting Qi circulation to remove stagnancy, expelling heat to cause laxation.

INDICATIONS

Stuffiness, fullness in the abdomen, abdominal pain with tenderness and guarding, loss of appetite, eructation with fetid odor, acid regurgitation, pus and blood in the stool, tenesmus, burning sensation in the anus, oliguria with deep colour, yellow and greasy tongue, slippery and rapid pulse due to food retention and stagnation of Qi.

DIRECTIONS

To be taken orally, 6~9g each time, twice a day.

PRECAUTION

For those with abdominal distension due to deficiency and constipation due to deficiency of YIN, it is not fit. And it is contraindicated in pregnant women.

100 KAIXIONG SHUNQI WAN （开胸顺气丸）

Pill for Relieving Stagnation and Smoothing Qi

PRINCIPAL INGREDIENTS

Dried green orange peel (Pericarpium Citri Reticulatae Viride), Malt (Fructus Hordei Germinatus), Licorice root (Radix Glycyrrhizae), Rhubarb (Radix et Rhizoma Rhei), Medicated leaven (Massa Medicata Fermentata), Bark of official magnolia (Cortex Magnoliae Officinalis), Chinese radish seed (Semen Raphani), Root of three-nerved Spicebush (Radix Linderae), Costusroot (Radix Saussureae Lappae), Fruit of hawthorn (Fructus Crataegi), Fruit of immature bitter orange (Fructus Aurantii Immaturus), Betel nut (Semen Arecae)

FUNCTIONS

Relieving stagnation of to smooth Qi circulation, promoting digestion to remove food retention.

INDICATIONS

Stuffiness, distension and pain in the abdomen, stomachache, eructation with fetid odor, acid regurgitation, loss of appetite, nausea, vomiting, pain relieved after vomiting, pus and blood in the stool, tenesmus, greasy tongue coating, slippery and wiry pulse due to stagnation of Qi and retention of food.

DIRECTIONS

To be taken orally, 6~9 g each time for adult, 2~3 times a day, and half of dosage for who is above seven.

PRECAUTION

It is contraindicated in pregnant women and patients with deficiency of Qi. And it is not fit for those with dyspepsia due to deficiency of the spleen and had symptom of loose stool.

101   ZHISHI XIAOPI WAN （枳实消痞丸）

Pill of Immature Bitter Orange for Disintegrating Masses and Relieving Stuffiness

PRINCIPAL INGREDIENTS

Fruit of immature bitter Orange (Fructus Aurantii Immaturus), Chinese goldthread (Rhizoma Coptidis), Bark of official magnolia (Cortex Magnoliae Officinalis), Large-headed atractylodes (Rhizoma Atractylodis Macrocephalae), Pinellia (Rhizoma Pinelliae), Malt (Fructus Hordei Germinatus), Tuckahoe (Poria), Licorice root (Radix Glycyrrhizae), Pilose asiabell root (Radix

Codonopsis Pilosulae), Dried ginger (Rhizoma Zingiberis)

FUNCTIONS

Disintegrating masses and relieving stuffiness, invigorating the spleen and regulating the stomach.

INDICATIONS

Stuffiness and fullness due to deficiency of the spleen and cold-heat twined, manifested as stuffiness and fullness in the upper abdomen, poor appetite, indigestion, lassitude, weakness, dyschesia, yellow and greasy tongue coating, or white and greasy tongue coating, and soft and floating pulse, or slippery and rapid pulse.

DIRECTIONS

To be taken orally, 9g each time for adult, three times a day, 6g each time for over seven; 3g for three to seven.

102 LIUQU CHA (六曲茶)

Tea with Medicated Leaven

PRINCIPAL INGREDIENTS

Medicated leaven (Massa Medicata Fermentata), Malt (Fructus Hordei Germinatus), Fruit of hawthorn (Fructus Crataegi), Pinellia (Rhizoma Pinelliae), Dahurian angelica (Radix Angelicae Dahuricae), Betel nut (Semen Arecae), Leaf of purple perilla (Folium Perillae), Chinese atractylodes (Rhizoma Atractylodis), Dried old orange peel (Pericarpium Citri Reticulatae), Tuckaohe (Poria), Licorice root (Radix Glycyrrhizae), Wrinkled gianthyssop (Herba Agastachis), Nutgrass flatsedge (Rhizoma Cyperi), Root of balloonflower (Radix Platycodi), Amomum fruit (Fructus Amomi), Round cardamom seed (Semen Cardamomi Rotundi), Bark of official magnolia (Cortex Magnoliae Officinalis)

FUNCTIONS

Invigorating the spleen to promote digestion and expelling cold.

INDICATIONS

Food retention manifested abdominal pain with tenderness and guarding, distension and fullness in the abdomen, eructation with fetid odor, nausea, vomiting, thick and greasy tongue coating, and wiry and slippery pulse; common cold shows headache, aversion to cold, nasal discharge, cough with white phlegm, floating and tight pulse, and white and greasy tongue coating.

DIRECTIONS

It can be taken as a tea, 1～2 piece each time, twice a day.

PRECAUTION

It is forbidden to take raw, cold, oily and greasy food.

103 MINDONG JIANQU（闽东建曲）

Jianqu from East of Fujian

PRINCIPAL INGREDIENTS

Amomum fruit (Fructus Amomi), Clove (Flos Syzygii Aromatici), Katsumadai seed (Semen Alpiniae Katsumadai), Rice sprout (Fructus Oryzae Ferminatus), Costusroot (Radix Saussureae Lappae), Malt (Fructus Hordei Germinatus), Spikenard (Rhizoma Nardostachyos), Licorice root (Radix Glycyrrhizae), Chinese mugwort leaf (Folium Atremisiae Argyi), Leaf of purple perilla (Folium Perillae), Wrinkled gianthyssop (Herba Agastachis), Resurrectionlily (Rhizoma Kaempferiae), Fruit of hawthorn (Fructus Crataegi), Fruit of immature bitter orange (Fructus Aurantii Immaturus), Tuckahoe (Poria), Lesser galangal (Rhizoma Alpiniae Officinarum), Schizonepeta (Herba Schizonepetae), Sweet wormwood

(Herba Artemisiae Chinghao), Evodia fruit (Fructus Evodiae), Notopterygium (Rhizoma Seu Radix Noto-pterygii), Citron (Fructus Citri Sarcodactylis), Dahurian angelica (Radix Angelicae Dahuricae), Pinellia (Rhizoma Pinelliae), Chinese atractylodes (Rhizoma Atractylodis), Paniculate swallowwort root (Radix Cynanchi Paniculati), Betel nut (Semen Arecae), Nutgrass flatsedge (Rhizoma Cyperi), Bark of official magnolia (cortex Magnoliae Officinalis), Dried old orange peel (Pericarpium Citri Reticulatae), Root of balloonflower (Radix Platycodi), Fruit of citron or trifoliate orange (Fructus Aurantii), Skullcap (Radix Scutellariae), Ledebouriella (Radix Ledebouriellae), Wheat flour Red rice (Monascus Purpureus), Herb of polygone (Herb Polygoni Hydropiperis)

FUNCTIONS

Warming the middle JIAO to expel cold, expelling wind to relieve exterior syndrome, and expelling wetness and heat in the summer.

INDICATIONS

Stomachache due to cold in the stomach, manifested as stomachache, aggravation from cold, distension and fullness in the abdomen, poor appetite, indigestion, or vomiting, diarrhea, white and greasy tongue coating, and wiry and slippery pulse; common cold due to exterior wind and cold, manifested as chill, fever, headache, pantagia, nasal discharge, cough with white and thin phlegm, white and greasy tongue coating, and floating; common cold due to wetness and heat in the summer shows headache, stuffiness and fullness in the chest, nausea, white and greasy tongue coating, and floating, soft and rapid pulse.

DIRECTIONS

To be taken as a tea, one piece each time, twice a day.

PRECAUTION

Patient, with deficiency of YIN and hyperactivity of fire, should be avoided to take.

104 SHUNQI XIAOSHI HUATAN WAN（顺气消食化痰丸）

Pill for Smoothing Qi, Promoting Digestion And Expelling Phlegm

PRINCIPAL INGREDIENTS

Pinellia （Rhiz oma Pinelliae）, Fruit of hawthorn (Fructus Crataegi), Jack-in-the-pulpit (Rhizoma Arisaematis), Medicated leaven (Massa Medicata Fermentata), Apricot (Semen Armeniacae Amarum), Root of kudzuvine (Radix Puerariae), Dried green orange peel (Pericarpium Citri Reticulatae), Malt (Fructus Hordei Germinatus), Fruit of purple perilla (Folium Perillae), Chinese radish seed (Semen Raphani), Nutgrass flatsedge (Rhizoma Cyperi), Dried old orange peel (Pericarpium Citri Reticulatae), Agalloch eaglewood (Lignum Aquilariae Resinatum), Ginger (Rhizoma Zingiberis Recens).

FUNCTIONS

Smoothing Qi, promoting digestion and expelling phlegm.

INDICATIONS

Food retention in the stomach and cough due to wetness and phlegm, manifested as stuffiness and fullness in the chest and abdomen, cough with copious and white phlegm, eructation with fetid odor, acid regurgitation, loose of appetite, or accompanying with nausea, vomiting, greasy tongue coating, and slippery pulse.

DIRECTIONS

To be taken orally, 6g each time, three

times a day.

PRECAUTION

It is forbidden to take raw, cold, oily and greasy food, and contraindicated in pregnant women.

I -6 Prescriptions for purging
泻下剂

105 GENGYI WAN (更衣丸)

Purgative Pill

PRINCIPAL INGREDIENTS

Aloe (Aloe), Cinnabar (Cinnabaris)

FUNCTIONS

Purging fire and promoting bowels movement.

INDICATIONS

Constipation accompanying with irritability with inclination to anger, insomnia, bitter mouth, conjunctivitis due to fire retained in the stomach and intestine.

DIRECTIONS

To be taken orally, 3g each time, 1 ~ 2 times a day for adult, half of dosage for child.

PRECAUTION

It is contraindicated in pregnant women.

And it is not fit for those are weak and senior.

106 QINGNING WAN （清宁丸）

Pill for Clearing away Heat and Purgation

PRINCIPAL INGREDIENTS

Rhubarb (Radix et Rhizoma Rhei), Bark of official magnolia (Cortex Magnoliae Officinalis), Dried old orange peel (Pericarpium Citri Reticulatae), Nutgrass flatsedge (Rhizoma Cyperi), Skullcap (Radix Scutellariae), Mung bean (Semen Phaseoli Aurei),Stick of Chinese scholartree (Ramulus Sophorae), Asiatic plantain (Herba Plantaginis), Large-headed atractylodes (Rhizoma Atractylodis Macrocephalae), Pinellia (Rhizoma Pinelliae),White mulberry Branch (Ramulus Mori), Black soybean (Glycine Max), Barley

FUNCTIONS

Purging fire to clear away heat, Promoting bowels movement and digestion to remove stagnancy.

INDICATIONS

Syndromes of heat retention in the stomach and intestine, or in the upper JIAO, or heat and wetness retained in the lower JIAO manifested as hard and dry stool, stuffiness and fullness with pain in the abdomen, dry mouth and lips, or thirst with inclination to drink, foul breath, fever with fidgeting, reddish complexion with conjunctivitis, sore throat, or oral ulceration, or oliguria with difficulty and pain in micturition, yellow tongue coating with reduced saliva, slippery and rapid pulse.

DIRECTIONS

To be taken orally, for honeyed pill, one pill each time, twice a day; for water-paste pill, 6g each time, twice a day.

PRECAUTION

It is not fit for senior, weak patient and pregnant women.

107 MAREN WAN （麻仁丸）

Pill with Hemp Seed

PRINCIPAL INGREDIENTS

Hemp seed (Fructus Cannabis), Root of herbaceous peony (Radix Paeoniae Alba), Apricot (Semen Armeniacae Amarum), Fruit of immature bitter orange (Fructus Aurantii Immaturus), Bark of official magnolia (Cortex Magnoliae Officinalis), Rhubarb (Radix et Rhizoma Rhei)

FUNCTIONS

Moistening the intestines to relieve constipation.

INDICATIONS

Constipation due to intestinal dryness, manifested as frequency of urination, dry stool.

DIRECTIONS

To be taken orally, 6~9g each time, twice.

PRECAUTION

It is contraindicated in pregnant women, and it can be a long-term taken for senior and weak patients.

108 ZHOUCHE WAN （舟车丸）

Pill for Relieving Ascites

PRINCIPAL INGREDIENTS

Morning glory seed (Semen Pharbitidis), Rhubarb (Radix et Rhizoma Rhei),Euphorbia root (Radix Knoxiae), kansui root (Radix Euphorbiae Kansui),Genkwa Flower (Flos Genkwa),Dried green orange peel (Citrus Reticulatae Viride), Dried old orange peel (Pericarpium Citri Reticulatae), Costusroot (Radix Saussureae Lappae), Betel nut (Semen Arecae),Calomel (Calomelas)

FUNCTIONS

Promoting Qi circulation and eliminating retained fluid, promoting bowels movement
and diuresis.

INDICATIONS

Excess syndrome of edema accompanying
with distension and swelling in the chest
and abdomen, dyspnea reddish complexion,
thirst, constipation, oliguria and deep,
rapid and forceful pulse.

DIRECTIONS

To be taken orally, 1.5 ~ 4.5g each time,
twice a day, or 3 ~ 6g each time, once a
day.

PRECAUTION

It is contraindicated in pregnant women and
weak one. It should be avoided to take salt
and soy sauce in 100 days, it can not be tak-
en with licorice root, and it can not be taken
for a long time.

109 WUREN RUNCHANG WAN （五仁润肠丸）

Pill with Five Kinds of Seeds for Causing
Laxation

PRINCIPAL INGREDIENTS

Peach kernel (Semen Persicae), Hemp seed
(Fructus Cannabis), Bunge cherry seed (Se-

men Pruni), Seed of oriental arborviate (Semen Biotae), Pine nut, Rehmannia (Radix Rehmanniae), Dried old orange peel (Pericarpium Citri Reticulatae), Chinese angelica (Radix Angelicae Sinensis), Saline cistanche (Herba Cistanchis), Rhubarb (Radix et Rhizoma Rhei)

FUNCTIONS

Nourishing YIN, enriching blood, moistening the intestines to relieve constipation, promoting digestion, and removing stagnancy.

INDICATIONS

Constipation, or hard stool, loss of appetite, distension in the abdomen due to deficiency of YIN, in the senior, or weak patient, or patient after labor and operation.

DIRECTIONS

To be taken orally, one pill each time, twice a day.

PRECAUTION

It is contraindicated in pregnant women.

I-7 Prescriptions for Relieving Diarrhea
止泻剂

110 SISHEN WAN (四神丸)

Pill with Four Mirraculou Drugs

PRINCIPAL INGREDIENTS

Saline cistanche (Herba Cistanchis), Evodia fruit (Fructus Forsythiae), Malaytea scurf-pea (Fructus Psoraleae), Chinese date (Fructus Ziziphi Jujubae), Fruit of Chinese magnoliavine Fructus Schisandrae), Ginger (Rhizoma Zingiberis Recens)

FUNCTIONS

Warming and tonifying the spleen and kidney to relieve diarrhea with astringency.

INDICATIONS

Diarrhea due to deficiency of the kidney-YANG manifested as diarrhea before dawn, abdominal pain with cold sensation, lassitude, weakness, loose stool, poor appetite, lumbago, cold limbs, pale tongue with white coating, and deep, slow and weak pulse.

DIRECTIONS

To be taken orally, 9g each time for adult, 1～2 times a day; half of dosage for child.

PRECAUTION

It is contraindicated in patients with diarrhea and abdominal pain caused by excessive heat.

111 GEGEN QINLIAN PIAN （葛根芩连片）

Tablet with Pueraria, Scutellaria and Coptis

PRINCIPAL INGREDIENTS

Root of kudszuvine （Radix Puerariae）, Skullcap （Radix Scutellariae）, Chinese goldthread （Rhizoma Coptidis）, Licorice root （Radix Glycyrrhizae）

FUNCTIONS

Clearing away heat, relieving exterior syndrome and diarrhea

INDICATIONS

Diarrhea due to exopathogenic heat invading the interior while the exterior symptoms remain unrelieved, manifested as fever, diarrhea, irritable hot sensation in the chest and abdomen, dry mouth, thirst, red tongue with yellow coating, and rapid pulse.

DIRECTIONS

To be taken orally, 3～4 tablets each time, three times a day.

PRECAUTION

It is contraindicated in diarrhea due to cold of deficiency.

112 XIANGLIAN WAN （香连丸）

Pill of Costusroot and Coptis

PRINCIPAL INGREDIENTS

Costusroot (Radix Saussureae Lappae), Chinese goldthread (Rhizoma Coptidis)

FUNCTIONS

Clearing away heat to detoxify, promoting Qi circulation to remove stagnancy.

INDICATIONS

Dysentery due to heat and wetness, manifested as dysentery, abdominal pain, vomiting, tenesmus, pus and blood in the stool. Enteritis and bacillary dysentery show above symptoms.

DIRECTIONS

To be taken orally, 3～6g each time, 2～3 times a day, child takes the half of dosage.

PRECAUTION

It is contraindicated in pregnant women, and spicy, oily and greasy food should be avoided to take.

113 KELISHA JIAONANG （克痢痧胶囊）

Capsule for Curing Dysentery

PRINCIPAL INGREDIENTS

Wildginger (Herba Asari), Dahurian angelica (Radix Angelicae Dahuricae), Alum (Alumen), Goose-will-not-eat herb (Herba Centipedae), Borneol (Borneolum Syntheticum）, Mirabilite (Mirabilitum), Chinese atractylodes (Rhizoma Atractylodis), Long pepper (Fructus Piperis Longi), Honeylocust fruit (Fructus Gleditsiae Abnormalis)

FUNCTIONS

Detoxifying, expelling filthiness, regulating Qi circulation and relieving diarrhea.

INDICATIONS

Abdominal pain accompanying with vomiting, diarrhea, or pus and blood in the stool, pale tongue with greasy coating, and deep and tight pulse caused by wind, cold, wetness and filthiness.

DIRECTIONS

To be taken orally, 2 capsules each time, three times a day.

PRECAUTION

It is contraindicated in pregnant women, and diarrhea and dysentery due to wetness and heat retention in the large intestine.

114　FUFANG HUANGLIANSU PIAN （复方黄连素片）

Compound Tablets of Berberine

PRINCIPAL INGREDIENTS

Berberine, Costusroot (Radix Saussureae

Lappae), Root of herbaceous peony (Radix
Paeoniae Alba), Evodia fruit (Fructus Evodiae)

FUNCTIONS

Clearing away heat from the intestines, promoting Qi circulation to relieve pain and diarrhea.

INDICATIONS

Acute enteritis manifested as diarrhea, yellow and watery stool, abdominal pain,
burning sensation in the anus, thirst, willing to take cold drinking, red tongue with
yellow and thick coating, and wiry and
rapid pulse; dysentery showed tenesmus,
pus and blood in the stool, pain around
navel, or accompanying with fever, red
tongue with yellow coating, and rapid
pulse.

DIRECTIONS

To be taken orally, 4 tablets each time,
four times a day.

PRECAUTION

It is forbidden to take spicy and greasy food
during the treatment. And it is contraindicated in enteritis and dysentery whose differentiation is deficient and cold.

Prescription for Expelling Phlegm，Arresting Cough and Relieving Asthma
祛痰–止咳–平喘剂

115 XIAO QINGLONG CHONGJI（小青龙冲剂）

Minor Infusion of Green Dragon

PRINCIPAL INGREDIENTS

Chinese ephedra (Herba Ephedrae)，Cassia (Ramulus Cinnamomi)，Root of herbaceous peony (Radix Paeoniae Alba)，Dried ginger (Rhizoma Zingiberis)，Wildginger (Herba Asari)，Pinellia (Rhizoma Pinelliae)，Fruit of Chinese magnoliavine (Fructus Schisandrae)，Licorice root (Radix Glycyrrhizae)

FUNCTIONS

Relieve exterior syndrome by means of inducing diaphoresis，removing fluid retention，arresting cough，relieving asthma.

INDICATIONS

Syndrome of phlegm with cold pathogen in the exterior，manifested as chill，fever，absence of perspiration，cough，asthma with watery，copious and white phlegm，which cause difficult to lie on one's back，edema in the face and lower limbs white，slippery and moist tongue coating，and floating tight pulse.

DIRECTIONS

To be taken orally, 1~2 pieces each time, 2~3 times a day for adult, half of dosage for child.

PRECAUTION

It should avoided to take raw and cold food, and take shelter from the wind and cold. And it is contraindicated in pregnant women.

116 ER CHEN WAN（二陈丸）

Pill with Two Old Drugs

PRINCIPAL INGREDIENTS

Pinellia (Rhizoma Pinelliae), Dried old orange peel (Pericarpium Citri Reticulatae), Tuckahoe (Poria), Licorice root (Radix Glycyrrhizae)

FUNCTIONS

Invigorating the spleen and promoting Qi circulation to expel phlegm and regulate the stomach.

INDICATIONS

Syndrome of wetness-phlegm, manifested as distension and fullness in the abdomen, loose of appetite, nausea, vomiting, cough with white phlegm, white and moist tongue coating, and slippery pulse.

DIRECTIONS

To be taken orally, 6 ～ 9g each time for adult, three times a day before meals.

PRECAUTION

It is contraindicated in dry-phlegm and phlegm with blood due to deficiency of lung-YIN.

117 TONGXUAN LIFEI WAN （通宣理肺丸）

Pill for Ventilating the Lung

PRINCIPAL INGREDIENTS

Chinese ephedra (Herba Ephedrae). Leaf of purule perilla (Folium Perillae). Root of purple-flowered peuce-danum （Radix Peucedani）. Apricot (Semen Armeniacae Amarum). Tuckahoe (Poria). Fruit of citron orange (Fructus Aurantii). Root of balloon-flower (Radix Platycodi). Dried old orange peel (Pericarpium Citri Reticulatae). Pinellia （Rhizoma Pinelliae）. Skullcap （Radix Scutellariae）. Licorice root （Radix Glycyrrhizae）

FUNCTIONS

Relieving exterior syndrome and expelling by means of inducing diaphoresis, relieving cough and expelling phlegm.

INDICATIONS

Aversion to cold, chill, headache, stuffy nose cough with white phlegm, perspiration, dyspnea, pantalgia, arthralgia, thin and white tongue coating, and floating and tight pulse.

DIRECTIONS

To be taken orally, two pills each time, 2~3 times a day, a half of dosage for child who is above seven years old, one third of dosage for child who is three to seven.

PRECAUTION

It is contraindicated in common cold due to wind-heat and cough due to deficiency of YIN. And raw, cold, stick and greasy food should be avoided to take.

118 XIAO KECHUAN （消咳喘）

Syrup for Relieving Cough and Asthma

PRINCIPAL INGREDIENTS

Daurian rhododendron leaf (Folium Rhododendri Daurici)

FUNCTIONS

Arresting cough, expelling phlegm, relieving asthma.

INDICATIONS

Cough, asthma, shortness of breath, even

being difficult to lie on one's back. Common cold, chronic bronchitis and pulmonary emphysema show above symptoms.

DIRECTIONS

To be taken orally, 7 ~ 10ml each time, three times a day.

PRECAUTION

It should be avoided to take spicy and irritant food.

119 FUFANG CHUANBEIJING PIAN（复方川贝精片）

Compound Tablet of Sichuan Fritillary Bulb

PRINCIPAL INGREDIENTS

Tendril-leaved fritillary bulb (Bulbus Fritillariae Cirrhosae), Chinese ephedra (Herba Ephedrae), Dried old orange peel (Pericarpium Citri Reticulatae), Pinellia (Rhizoma Pinelliae), Root of the narrow-leaved polygala (Radix Polygalae), Root of balloonflower (Radix Platycodi), Fruit of Chinese magnoliavine (Fructus Schisandrae), Licorice root (Radix Glycyrrhizae)

FUNCTIONS

Moisturizing the lung and expelling phlegm to arrest cough and relieve asthma.

INDICATIONS

Cough with copious, white and watery phlegm, asthma, shortness of breath, stuffiness and fullness in the chest and abdomen, pale tongue with white and moist coating, or thick and greasy coating, and soft and slippery pulse.

DIRECTIONS

To be taken orally, 3~6 tablets each time for adult, three times a day; a half of dosage for who is above seven; one third of dosage for who is three to seven.

PRECAUTION

To take shelter from the wind and cold during the treatment.

120 QINGQI HUATAN WAN (清气化痰丸)

Pill for Clearing Heat and Expelling Phlegm

PRINCIPAL INGREDIENTS

Jack-in-the-pulpit (Rhizoma Arisaematis), Skullcap (Radix Scutellariae), Seed of mongolian snakegourd (Semen Trichosanthis), Dried old orange peel (Pericarpium Citri Reticulatae), Apricot (Semen Armeniacae Amarum), Tuckahoe (Poria), Fruit of immature bitter orange (Fructus Aurantii Immaturus), Pinellia (Rhizoma Pinelliae)

FUNCTIONS

Clearing away heat from the lung, promoting Qi circulation and expelling.

INDICATIONS

Cough, asthma with phlegm due to phlegm and heat in the lung, manifested as cough with yellow and stick phlegm, stuffiness and fullness in the chest, thirst, or hard stool, fever, even cough and asthma with pain in the chest, blood in the phlegm, red tongue with yellow and greasy coating, and slippery pulse.

DIRECTIONS

To be taken orally, 6～9g each time, twice a day.

PRECAUTION

It is contraindicated in pregnant women, and patients, who is weak, with loose stool.

121 LINGYANG QINGFEI WAN (羚羊清肺丸)

Pill with Antelope Horn for Clearing away Heat from Lung

PRINCIPAL INGREDIENTS

Antelope horn (Cornu Antelopis), Fritillary

bulb (Bulbus Fritillariae Thunbergii),Dyers
woad leaf (Folium Isatidis), Dried root of
rehmannia (Radix Rehmannia), Root-bark
of white mulberry (Cortex Mori Radicis),
Root of Zhejiang figwort (Radix Scutellariae Barbatae), Licorice root (Radix Glycyrrhizae),Stem of noble dendrobium (Herba Dendrobrii), Capejasmine (Fructus Gardeniae), Dried old orange peel (Pericarpium
Citri Reticulatae), Honeysuckle flower
(Flos Lonicerae),Apricot (Semen Armeniacae Amarum),Root of balloonflower (Radix
Platycodi), Tinospora (Radix Tinosprae),
Peppermint oil (Oleum Menthae),Flower of
loquat (Folium Eriobotryae), Lucid asparagus (Radix Asparagi), Root of Chinese trichosanthes (Radix Trichosanthis), Dyers
woad root (Radix Isatidis),Skullcap (Radix
Scutellariae), Root of purple-flowered
peucedanum (Radix Peucedani), Root-bark
of peony (Cortex Moutan Radicis),Rhubarb
(Radix et Rhizoma Rhei), Tuber of dwarf
lilyturf (Radix Ophiopogonis)

FUNCTIONS

Clearing away heat from the lung, arresting
cough, expelling phlegm, detoxifying, relieving sore throat, nourishing YIN, and

moistening the lung.

INDICATIONS

Affection due to exogenous pathogen with over abundance of heat located at the lung. manifested as cough with yellow phlegm. fever. pantagia. headache. thirst. sore throat. epistaxis. hemoptysis. red tongue with yellow coating. and floating and rapid pulse. or wiry and rapid pulse.

DIRECTIONS

To be taken orally. one pill each time for adult. three times a day; the half of pill for child who is over seven; and one third of pill for who is three to seven.

PRECAUTION

It is forbidden to take spicy food. and contraindicated in pregnant women.

122 SHEDAN CHENPI MO (蛇胆陈皮末)

Powder with Snake Bill and Dried Old Orange Peel

PRINCIPAL INGREDIENTS

Snake bile Fried old orange peel (Pericarpium Citri Reticulatae). Cinnabar (Cinnabaris). Larva of a silkworm with batrytis (Bombyx Batryticatus). Amber (Succinum). Earth-worm (Lumbricus)

FUNCTIONS

Clearing away heat, expelling phlegm, calming down the interior-wind, and relieving the muscular spasm.

INDICATIONS

High fever, cough with yellow, thick and stick phlegm, convulsion, coma due to syndrome of wind-phlegm and heat, especially in the child.

DIRECTIONS

To be taken orally, 0.3~0.6g each time, 2~3 times a day.

PRECAUTION

It is contraindicated in pregnant women.

123 SHEDAN CHUANBEI SAN （蛇胆川贝散）

Powder of Snake Bile and Sichuan Fritillary Bulb

PRINCIPAL INGREDIENTS

Snake bile, Tendril-leaved fritillary bulb (Bulbus Fritillariae Cirrhosae)

FUNCTIONS

Clearing away heat, expelling wind and phlegm, arresting cough.

INDICATIONS

Cough due to phlegm and heat retained in the lung, manifested as fever, sore throat,

cough with yellow, stick and thick phlegm,
red tongue with yellow and greasy coating,
and slippery and rapid pulse.

DIRECTIONS

To be taken orally, 0. 3~0. 6g each time, 2
~3 times a day.

PRECAUTION

It should be avoided to take for loose stool
due to deficiency of the spleen.

124 JUHONG WAN (橘红丸)

Pill with Tangerine Peel

PRINCIPAL INGREDIENTS

Tangerine peel (Exocarpium Citri
Grandis), Peel of mongolian snakegourd
(Pericarpium Trichosanthis), Dried old or-
ange peel (Pericarpium Citri Reticulatae),
Plaster stone (Gypsum Fibrosum), Apricot
(Semen Armeniacae Amarum), Fritillary
bulb (Bulbus Fritillariae Thunbergii),
Pinellia (Rhizoma Pinelliae), Tuckahoe
(Poria), Root of balloonflower (Radix
Platycodi), Fruit of purple perilla (Fructus
Perillae), Tatarian aster (Radix Asteris),
Common coltsfoot flower (Flos Farfarae),
Rehmannia (Radix Rehmanniae), Tuber of
dwarf lilyturf (Radix Ophiopogonis),

Licorice root （Radix Glycyrrhizae）

FUNCTIONS

Clearing away heat and expelling phlegm

INDICATIONS

Cough due to heat and phlegm retained in the lung, manifested as cough with copious, yellow, stick and thick phlegm, stuffiness, asthma, red tongue with yellow and greasy coating, and slippery.

DIRECTIONS

To be taken orally, one pill each time for adult, and two pills each time for severe one, twice a day.

PRECAUTION

It is forbidden to take spicy, oily and greasy food.

125　DITAN WAN （涤痰丸）

Pill for Expelling Phlegm

PRINCIPAL INGREDIENTS

Morning glory seed （Semen Pharbitidis）, Rhubarb （Radix et Rhizoma Rhei）,Skullcap （Radix Scutellariae）

FUNCTIONS

Clearing away heat and expelling stubborn phlegm.

INDICATIONS

Syndrome of heat and stubborn phlegm, manifested as insanity, palpitation, or cough and asthma with stick phlegm, or dizziness, coma, accompanying with flushed complexion, conjunctivitis, constipation, yellow and greasy tongue coating, and slippery, rapid and forceful pulse.

DIRECTIONS

To be taken orally, 6g each time for adult, once a day, and a half of dosage for above seven, one third of dosage for three to seven.

PRECAUTION

It is contraindicated in pregnant women, and deficient one.

126 JI SU WAN (鸡苏丸)

Pill with Purple Perilla for Relieving Asthma

PRINCIPAL INGREDIENTS

Chinese ephedra (Herba Ephedrae), Apricot (Semen Armeniacae Amarum), Plaster stone (Gypsum Fibrosum), Licorice root (Radix Glycyrrhizae), Skullcap (Radix Scutellariae), Seed of pepperweed tansymustard (Semen Lepidii seu Descurainiae), Root-bark of white mulberry (Cortex Mori

Radicis), Birthwort (Fructus Aristolochiae),Lucid asparagus (Radix Asparagi), Tuber of dwarf lilyturf (Radix Ophiopogonis), Beishashen (Radix Glehniac), Fruit of Chinese magnoliavine (Fructus Schisandrae), Root of merbaceous peony (Radix Paeoniae Alba), Rhizome old wind-weed (Rhizoma Anemarrhenae), Lily bulb (Bulbus Lilii), Tatarian aster (Radix Asteris), Common coltsfoot flower (Flos Farfarae), Seed of mongolian snakegourd (Semen Trichosanthis), Root of balloonflower (Radix Platycodi), Root of purple-flowered peucedanum (Radix Peucedani), Leaf of purple perilla (Folium Perillae), Tangerine peel (Exocarpium Citri Grandis), Pinellia (Rhizoma Pinelliae), Dried old orange peel (Pericarpium Citri Reticulatae), Root of the narrow -leaved polygala (Radix Polygalae), Ginger (Rhizoma Zingiberis Recens), Chinese date (Fructus Ziziphi Jujubae)

FUNCTIONS

Clearing away heat, relieving asthma, moistening dryness, arresting cough, expelling phlegm, disintegrating masses and relieving stuffiness.

INDICATIONS

Syndrome of cough and asthma due to heat retained in the lung. due to dryness. or due to deficiency of YIN. manifested as cough. asthma. dyspnea. nares flaring. red tongue with yellow coating. and rapid pulse. or cough with stick phlegm. dry throat and nasal cavity. or cough with bloody phlegm. hectic fever. flushed zygomatic region. night sweat. stuffiness and fullness in the chest. red tongue. and thread and rapid pulse.

DIRECTIONS

To be taken orally. 3～6g each time. 2～3 times a day.

PRECAUTION

It is contraindicated in cough and asthma due to wetness-phlegm. and phlegm and cold retained in the lung.

127 QIULI GAO（秋梨膏）

Pear Syrup

PRINCIPAL INGREDIENTS

Ussurian pear（Pyrus Ussurian Maxin）. Fritillary bulb（Bulbus Fritillariae Thunbergii）. Tuber of dwarf lilyturf（Radix Ophiopogonis）. Green radish. Fresh lotus rhizome（Rhizoma Nelumbinis）

FUNCTIONS

Nourishing YIN to promote the production of fluid, expelling phlegm to relieve cough.

INDICATIONS

Cough due to heat retained in the lung with deficiency of YIN, manifested as dry cough, shortness of breath, or cough with less stick phlegm, or bloody phlegm, dry mouth and throat, hoarseness, feverish sensation in the palms and soles, irritability, night sweat, flushed zygomatic region, hectic fever, red tongue with less fluid, and thread and rapid pulse.

DIRECTIONS

To be taken orally, 15g each time, twice a day.

PRECAUTION

It is forbidden to take spicy food.

128 YI XIAN WAN (医痫丸)

Pill for Epilepsy

PRINCIPAL INGREDIENTS

Baifuzi (Rhizoma Typhonii), Jack-in-the-pulpit (Rhizoma Arisaematis), Pinellia (Rhizoma Pinelliae), Honeylocust fruit (Fructus Gleditsiae Abnormalis), Larva of a silkworm with batrytis (Bombyx Batryticatus), Black-snake (Zaocys), Centipede (Scolopendra), Scorpion (Scorpio), Cinnabar (Cinnabaris), Alum (Alumen), Realgar (Realgar)

FUNCTIONS

Calming down interior-wind and expelling to arrest convulsion.

INDICATIONS

Epilepsy due to liver-wind and phlegm, manifested as sudden loss of consciousness, convulsion of extremities during a fit of epilepsy, trismus, eyeballs turing upward, foam in the mouth, white and greasy tongue coating, and wiry and slippery pulse.

DIRECTIONS

To be taken orally, 3g each time for adult, twice a day, and a half of dosage for who is five to ten.

PRECAUTION

It is forbidden to take sweet, oily and greasy food,, and contraindicated in pregnant women.

129 MENGSHI GUNTAN WAN (礞石滚痰丸)

Pill with Phlogopite for Removing Phlegm

PRINCIPAL INGREDIENTS

Phlogopite (Lapis Micae Aureus), Rhubarb

(Radix et Rhizoma Rhei), Skullcap (Radix Scutellariae), Agalloch eaglewood (Lignum Aquilariae Resinatum)

FUNCTIONS

Removing phlegm, dispersing the accumulation and purging the fire to cause laxation.

INDICATIONS

Depressive psychosis, mania, coma, vertigo, asthma, cough, ect. due to stubborn phlegm and heat, manifested as irritability, stuffiness and fullness in the chest, copious phlegm, constipation, deep and red tongue with yellow and greasy coating, slippery, rapid and forceful pulse.

DIRECTIONS

To be taken orally before meal, 9g each time, 1~2 times a day.

PRECAUTION

It is contraindicated in pregnant women, senior and weak one.

130 QINGXIN GUNTAN WAN (清心滚痰丸)

Pill for Clearing away Heat from Heart and Removing Phlegm

PRINCIPAL INGREDIENTS

Pholgopite (Lapis Micae Aureus), Agalloch

eaglewood (Lignum Aquilariae Resinatum), Skullcap (Radix Scutellariae), Rhubarb (Radix et Rhizoma Rhei), Honeylocust fruit (Fructus Gleditsiae Abnormalis), Gansui (Radix Euphorbiae Kansui), Morning glory seed (Semen Pharbitidis), Musk (Moschus), Borneol (Borneolum Syntheticum), Cow-bezoar (Calculus Bovis), Cinnabar (Cinnabaris), Pearl (Marapax Eretmochelydis), Long-noded pit viper (Ancistrodon Acutus), Rhinoceros horn (Cornu Rhinoceri), Antelope horn (Cornu Antelopis), Bark of Chinese cassia tree (Cortex Cinnamomi), Ginseng (Radix Ginseng)

FUNCTIONS

Expelling phlegm to causing resuscitation and tranquilizing interior wind to relieve convulsion.

INDICATIONS

Depressive psychosis, mania and epilepsy due to stubborn phlegm accompanying with heat, manifested as emotional depression, dementia, constant scolding and beating, irritability, flushed face, blood-shot eyes, red tongue with greasy coating, and wiry, slippery and forceful pulse.

DIRECTIONS

To be taken orally, one pill each time, twice a day.

PRECAUTION

It is contraindicated in pregnant women, patient who is weak, and phlegm syndrome except stubborn phlegm accompanying with excessive heat.

131 ZHISOU WAN（止嗽丸）

Pill for Relieving Cough

PRINCIPAL INGREDIENTS

Tatarian aster (Radix Asteris), White swallowwort (Rhizoma Cynanchi Vincetoxici), Stemona (Radix Stemonae), Dried old orange peel (Pericarpium Citri Reticulatae), Jingjie (Herba Schizonepetae), Root of balloonflower (Radix Platycodi), Licorice root (Radix Glycyrrhizae)

FUNCTIONS

Ventilating the lung to relieve cough.

INDICATIONS

Cough with pharyngeal parenthesis, or slight chill, nasal discharge, heavy limbs, white and thin tongue coating, and floating pulse due to the lung Qi inhibited caused by invaded wine.

To be taken orally before meals, 20 ~ 40 pills each time, 2~3 times a day.

PRECAUTION

Since this recipe is warm and dry, it is contraindicated in cough with deficiency of YIN.

132 ERMU NINGSOU WAN (二母宁嗽丸)

Pill with Fritillary Bulb and Rhizome of Wind-weed for Relieving Cough

PRINCIPAL INGREDIENTS

Fritillary bulb (Bulbus Fritillarae Thunbergii), Rhizome of wind-weed (Rhizoma Anemarrhenae), Plaster stone (Gypsum Fibrosum), Skullcap (Radix Scutellariae), Capejasmine (Fructus Gardeniae), Rootbark of white mulberry (Cortex Mori Radicis), Seed of mongolian snakegourd (Semen Trichosanthis), Dried old orange peel (Pericarpium Citri Reticulatae), Tuckahoe (Poria), Fruit of Chinese magnoliavine (Fructus Schisandrae), Fruit of immature bitter orange (Fructus Aurantii Immaturus), Licorice root (Radix Glycyrrhizae)

FUNCTIONS

Clearing away heat from the lung and

moistening the lung to relieve cough.

INDICATIONS

Cough caused by dryness and heat in the lung, manifested as cough with less, yellow and thick phlegm, or dry cough, fullness and stuffiness in the chest, dyspnea, dry mouth and throat, hoarseness, red tongue with yellow and thin coating, or without coating, and thread pulse, or thread and rapid pulse.

DIRECTIONS

To be taken orally before meal, 9g each time, twice a day.

PRECAUTION

This recipe should be administered carefully to patient with deficiency of kidney and Qi.

133 QIONGYU GAO (琼玉膏)

Jade Extract

PRINCIPAL INGREDIENTS

Rehmannia (Radix Rehmanniae), Tuckaohe (Poria), Dangshen (Radix Codonopsis Pilosulae), Honey (Mel)

FUNCTIONS

Nourishing YIN, moistening the lung, and tonifying and regulating the spleen and stomach.

INDICATIONS

Cough due to deficiency of the lung and stomach, manifested as cough with less phlegm, dyspnea, dry mouth and throat, eructation, deep and red tongue with less coating, thread and rapid pulse.

DIRECTIONS

To be taken orally, 15g each time, three time a day.

PRECAUTION

This should be administered carefully to patient exterior syndrome and loose stool due to deficiency of the spleen, and it is forbidden to take spicy food.

134 GEJIE DINGCHUAN WAN（蛤蚧定喘丸）

Pill with Gecko for Relieving Asthma

PRINCIPAL INGREDIENTS

Gecko (Gecko), Seed of mongolian snakegourd (Semen Trichosanthis), Chinese ephedra (Herba Ephedrae), Tatarian aster (Radix Asteris), Turtle shell (Carapax Trionycis), Skullcap (Radix Scutellariae), Licorice root (Radix Glycyrrhizae), Tuber of dwarf lilyturf (Radix Ophiopogonis), Chinese goldthread (Rhizoma Coptidis), Lily bulb (Bulbus Lilii), Fruit of purple perilla (Fructus Perillae), Apricot (Semen Armeniacae Amarum), Cinnabar (Cinnabaris), Plaster stone (Gypsum Fibrosum)

FUNCTIONS

Moistening the lung, tonifying the kidney, relieving asthma, arresting cough, clearing away heat and expelling phlegm.

INDICATIONS

Cough and asthma due to deficiency of lung, spleen and kidney accompanying with dryness-phlegm, manifested as cough with less phlegm, asthma, dyspnea, shortness of breath, weakness, lassitude of limbs, dry mouth and throat, red tongue, and thread rapid pulse, or deep and thread pulse.

DIRECTIONS

To be taken orally, one pill each time, twice a day.

PRECAUTION

It is contraindicated in cough and asthma caused by wind and cold, and excessive heat.

135 DINGCHUAN GAO（定喘膏）

Plaster for Relieving Asthma

PRINCIPAL INGREDIENTS

Burnt hair (Crinis Carbonisatus), Onion

Mankshood (Radix Aconiti Praeparata),
Dried ginger (Rhizoma Zingiberis), Jack-in-
the-pulpit (Rhizoma Arisaematis)

FUNCTIONS

Expelling cold, removing phlegm, and regulating Qi circulation to relieve asthma.

INDICATIONS

Asthma due to cold and phlegm retention in
the lung, manifested as cough with copious, white and thin phlegm, stuffiness and
fullness in the chest, asthma, dyspnea,
pale tongue with white and greasy coating,
and wiry and slippery pulse, or soft, floating and slow plus.

DIRECTIONS

To be used externally, stuck a piece of
medicine on the lung shu every time.

PRECAUTION

It should take shelter from the wind and
cold, and avoid to take raw and cold.

136 HAN CHUAN WAN (寒喘丸)

Pill for Asthma due to Cold

PRINCIPAL INGREDIENTS

Blackberry lily (Rhizoma Belamcandae),
Chinese ephedra (Herba Ephedrae), Widgin-
ger (Herba Asari), Dried ginger (Rhizoma

Zingiberis), Common coltsfoot flower (Flos Farfarae), Pinellia (Rhizoma Pinelliae), Tatarian aster (Radix Asteris), Fruit of Chinese magnoliavine (Fructus Schisandrae), Chinese date (Fructus Ziziphi Jujubae)

FUNCTIONS

Warming the lung, expelling phlegm, arresting cough, and relieving asthma.

INDICATIONS

Cough and asthma with copious, white and thin phlegm, dyspnea with wheezing sound in throat, pale tongue with white and moist coating, and floating pulse due to wind-cold and phlegm retention in the lung.

DIRECTIONS

To be taken orally, 3~6g each time, twice a day.

PRECAUTION

This recipe can not be taken for a long time as it is warm and dry in nature. It is contraindicated in patient with deficiency of YIN and excess heat retention in the lung, and it is forbidden to take raw and cold food.

137 HEI XI DAN （黑锡丹）

Black Tin Pill

PRINCIPAL INGREDIENTS

Black Tin Sulphur (Sulfur), Agalloch eagle-wood (Lignum Aquilariae Resinatum), Malaytea scurfpea (Fructus Psoraleae), Costusroot (Radix Saussureae Lappae), Common fennel (Fructus Foeniculi), Nutmeg (Semen Myristicae), Actinolite (Actinolitum), Calabash gourd (Pericarpium Lagenariae), Chinaberry fruit (Fructus Meliae Toosendan), Mankshood (Radix Aconiti Praeparata), Bark of Chinese cassia tree (Cortex Cinnamomi)

FUNCTIONS

Warming and tonifying the kidney to maintain normal inspiration, expelling cold and phlegm regulating Qi circulation to relieve asthma.

INDICATIONS

Asthma caused by deficiency of YANG and excessive YIN, manifested as asthma and dyspnea with wheezing sound in the throat, cold limbs with spontaneous perspiration, pale tongue with white coating, and deep and thread pulse.

DIRECTIONS

To be taken orally with ginseng tea, 6g

each time.

PRECAUTION

This recipe can be taken for two to three times, and it is contraindicated in pregnant women and patient with the deficiency of lower JIAO since it is heavy, warm and dry in the nature.

138   XINGSU ZHIKE CHONGJI (杏苏止咳冲剂)

Infusion with Apricot and Purple Perilla for Arresting Cough

PRINCIPAL INGREDIENTS

Apricot (Semen Armeniacae Amarum), Leaf of purple perilla (Folium Perillae), Root of balloonflower (Radix Platycodi), Dried old orange peel (Pericarpium Citri Reticulatae), Root of purple-flowered peucedanum (Radix Peucedani), Licorice root (Radix Glycyrrhizae)

FUNCTIONS

Expelling wind and cold, ventilating to resolve phlegm retention.

INDICATIONS

Common cold and cough due to wind and cold retention in the lung, manifested as stuffy nose with nasal discharge, pharyngeal paraesthesia, cough with white and thin phlegm, white and moist tongue coating, and floating pulse, or tight pulse.

DIRECTIONS

To infuse the medicine, one pack each time, three times a day.

PRECAUTION

It should be avoided to take raw, cold, oily and greasy food.

139 SHEDAN CHUANBEI YE (蛇胆川贝液)

Liquid with Snake Bile and Sichuan Fritillary Bulb

PRINCIPAL INGREDIENTS

Tendril-leaved fritillary bulb (Bulbus Fritillariae Cirrhosae), Apricot (Semen Armeniacae Amarum), Honey (Mel), Peppermint oil (Oleum Menthae), Snake bile

FUNCTIONS

Clearing away heat, moistening the lung, and expelling phlegm to relieve cough.

INDICATIONS

Syndrome of heat retention in the lung, manifested as restless cough with copious, yellow, thick and stick phlegm, dyspnea, or acompanying with fever, slight chill, yellow tongue coating, and rapid pulse, or floating and rapid pulse.

DIRECTIONS

To be taken orally, one bottle (10ml) each time, twice a day

PRECAUTION

This recipe should be administered carefully to cough caused by cold.

I -9 Prescriptions for Warming the Interior
温里剂

140 FUZI LIZHONG WAN（附子理中丸）

Pill with Mankshood for Regulating the Function of Middle JIAO

PRINCIPAL INGREDIENTS

Mankshood （Radix Aconiti Praeparata）, Dangshen （Radix Codonopsis Pilosulae）, Large-headed atractylodes （Rhizoma Atractylodis Macrocephalae）, Dried ginger （Rhizoma Zingiberis）, Licorice root （Radix Glycyrrhizae）

FUNCTIONS

Warming middle JIAO, expelling cold and tonifying the spleen and stomach.

INDICATIONS

Syndrome of deficiency of the spleen and cold in the spleen and stomach, manifested as stomachache and abdominal pain with cold sensation and predilection for warmth and pressure by hand, vomiting, watery diarrhea, poor appetite, cold limbs, lassitude, weakness, pale tongue with white coating, deep, and thread and weak pulse, or deep and slow pulse.

DIRECTIONS

To be orally before meals, one pill each time, 2~3 times a day.

PRECAUTION

It is contraindicated in pregnant women.

141 LIANG FU WAN （良附丸）

Pill of Lesser Galangal and Nutgrass Flatsedge

PRINCIPAL INGREDIENTS

Lesser galangal (Rhizoma Alpiniae Officinarum), Nutgrass flatsedge （Rhizoma Cyperi)

FUNCTIONS

Warming the middle JIAO, expelling cold and promoting Qi circulation to relieve pain, dispersing the depressed liver-Qi and regulating the menstruation.

INDICATIONS

Stomachache with cold sensation, vomiting, eructation, distension and pain in chest, breast and hypochondrium with aggravation from being angry, pain and distension in the lower abdomen occurring with menstrual cycle, which can be relieved by warmth and pressing, pale tongue with white coating, and deep and wiry pulse due to liver-Qi stagnated and cold retained in the channel.

DIRECTIONS

To be taken orally, 3~6g each time, twice a day.

PRECAUTION

It is forbidden to be angry and catch cold, and it is contraindicated in patient with fire and Qi stagnated in the liver and stomach or bleeding.

142   NUAN Qi GAO（暖脐膏）

Plaster for Warming Navel

PRINCIPAL INGREDIENTS

Chinese angelica（Radix Angelicae Sinensis）, Dahurian angelica（Radix Angelicae Dahuricae）, Costusroot（Radix Saussureae Lappae）, Root of three-nerved spicebush（Radix Linderae）, Common fennel（Fructus Foeniculi）, Truestar anisetree（Fructus Il-

licii Veri）, Nutgrass flatsedge （Rhizoma
Cyperi）, Olibanum （Resina Boswelliae Car-
terii）, Common myrrh tree （Commiphora
Myrrha）, Clove （Flos Syzygii Aromatici）,
Ark of Chinese cassia tree （Cortex Cin-
namomi）, Agalloch eaglewood （Lignum
Aquilariae Resinatum）, Nusk （Moschus）

FUNCTIONS

Warming the navel, expelling cold, promoting Qi circulation and relieving pain.

INDICATIONS

Syndrome of deficiency of the spleen and
kidney, and excessive cold in the body,
manifested as cold limbs, pale complexion,
soreness and cold sensation in the waist and
knees, loose stool, or diarrhea before
dawn, copious, white and thin leukorrhagia, pale and enlarged tongue with white
and moist coating, and deep and weak
pulse.

DIRECTIONS

To be used externally, and stuck it on the
navel and abdomen.

PRECAUTION

It is contraindicated in pregnant women.

143 PING WEI WAN （平胃丸）

Peptic Pill

PRINCIPAL INGREDIENTS

Chinese atractylodes (Rhizoma Atracty-lodis), Bark of official magnolia (Cortex Magnoliae Officinalis), Dried old orange peel (Pericarpium Citri Reticulatae), Ginger (Rhizoma Zingiberis Recens), Chinese date (Fructus Aiziphi Jujubae), Licorice root (Radix Glycyrrhzae)

FUNCTIONS

Eliminating wetness and invigorating the spleen.

INDICATIONS

Stuffiness and fullness in the chest and abdomen, loose of appetite, tasteless, lassitude, sleepiness, heavy legs, loose stool, nausea, vomiting, white and greasy tongue coating, and slippery pulse due to wetness retention in the spleen and stomach.

DIRECTIONS

To be taken orally, 6～12g each time, three times a day.

PRECAUTION

It is contraindicated in pregnant women and patient with syndrome of deficiency and heat.

144 ZHOUSHI HUISHENG DAN (周氏回生丹)

Zhou's Pill for Rescuing Life

PRINCIPAL INGREDIENTS

Sandal wood (Lignum Santali), Musk (Moschus), Agalloch eagle wood (Lignum Aquilariae Resinatum), Costusroot (Radix Saussureae Lappae), Lilac (Flos Syzygii), Borneol (Borneolum Syntheticum), Realgar (Realgar), Euphorbia root (Radix Knoxiae), Edible tulip (Bulbus Cremastrae), Moleplant seed (Semen Euphorbiae Lathyridis), Cinnabar (Cinnabaris), Licorice root (Radix Glycyrrhizae), Chinese gall (Galla Chinensis), Medicated leaven (Massa Medicata Fermentata)

FUNCTIONS

Expelling wetness and cold in the summer, detoxifying, expelling filthiness, eliminating wetness and relieving pain.

INDICATIONS

Cholera, vomiting, wary diarrhea, abdominal colic, stuffiness and fullness in the chest and upper abdomen, cold limbs, cramp, white and greasy tongue coating, and floating, soft and rapid pulse. Cholera, food poisoning, acute gastroenteritis show above symptoms.

DIRECTIONS

To be taken orally, 10 pills each time, twice a day.

PRECAUTION

It is contraindicated in pregnant women.

145 DINGGUI SAN（丁桂散）

Powder of Clove and Bark of Chinese Cassia Tree

PRINCIPAL INGREDIENTS

Bark of Chinese cassia tree (Cortex Cinnamomi), Clove (Flos Syzygii Aromatici)

FUNCTIONS

Warming Yang to expelling cold, promoting Qi circulation to relieve pain.

INDICATIONS

Abdominal pain and lumbago relieved by warming, cold limbs, aversion to cold, vomiting, distension in the abdomen, pale complexion, loose stool, pale tongue with white coating, and deep and thread pulse due to infection of cold and wind, or deficiency and cold in the stomach.

DIRECTIONS

To be taken orally, 3g each time, three times a day.

It is forbidden to take raw and cold food, and patient should be avoided to catch wind and cold.

146 SHIXIANG NUANQI GAO (十香暖脐膏)

Plaster with Ten Kinds of Fragrant Medicine for Warming Navel

PRINCIPAL INGREDIENTS

Clove (Flos Syzygii Aromatici), Truestar anisetree (Fructus Illicii Veri), Root of three-nerved spicebush (Radix Linderae), Common fennel (Fructus Foeniculi), Chinese angelica (Radix Angelicae Sinensis), Bark of Chinese cassia tree (Cortex Cinnamomi), Agalloch eaglewood (Lignum Aquilariae Resinatum), Olibanum (Resina Boswelliae Carterii)

FUNCTIONS

Warming abdomen to expel cold and promoting Qi circulation to relieve pain.

INDICATIONS

Abdominal pain with aggravation from cold and relieved by warming, chill, aversion to cold, cold limbs, loose stool, diarrhea, indigestion, lassitude in the waist and knees, pale tongue with white coating, and deep and thread pulse caused by excess cold retention in the abdomen.

DIRECTIONS

External application, to be stuck on the navel and abdomen, or on where is pain.

PRECAUTION

It is forbidden to use while the location is erythralgia with edema and hot sensation.

I -10 Prescriptions for Regulating the Flow of Qi
理气剂

147 XIAOYAO WAN（逍遥丸）

Ease Pill

PRINCIPAL INGREDIENTS

Bupleurum root (Radix Bupleuri), Chinese angelica root（Radix Angelicae Sinensis）, White peony root（Radix Paeoniae Alba）, Bighead atractylodes rhizome （Rhizoma AtractylodisMacrocephalae）, Poria (Poria), Liquorice（Radix Glycyrrhizae）, Peppermint (Herba Menthae)

FUNCTIONS

Soothing the liver, strengthening the spleen, and nourishing the blood to restore normal menstruation.

INDICATIONS

Stagnation of the liver-Qi and deficiency of the spleen manifested as distension in the chest and hypochondrium, dizziness, anorexia, loose stool, irregular menstruation and others.

DIRECTIONS

To be taken orally, 6～9 each time, 1～2 times a day.

PRECAUTION

The recipe is contraindicated in patients with cold limbs due to excess of heat which is caused by stagnation of Yin-Yang.

148　JIA WEI XIAOYAO WAN（加味逍遥丸）

Modified Ease Pill

PRINCIPAL INGREDIENTS

Bupleurum root (Radix Bupleuri). Chinese angelica root (Radix Angelicae Sinen is). White peony root (Radix Paeoniae Alba). Moutan bark (Cortex Moutan Radicis). Big-head atractylodes rhizome (Rhizoma Atracty-lodis Macrocephalae). Poria (Poria). Capejesmine (Fructus Gardeniae). Peppermint (Herba Menthae). Liguorice root (Radix Glycyrrhizae)

FUNCTIONS

Reinforcing function of the spleen to dispel dampness, removing evil heat and soothing the liver

INDICATIONS

Optic atrophy, retinitis centralis serosa, nonicterohepatitis, acute gastritis, gastro-duodenal ulcer. Pertain to the syndrome of stagnation of the liver-Qi and deficiency of blood and subsequent fire-transmission, with the symptoms of include dizziness and feeling of fullness in the eyes, mental depression, hypochondriac pain, red tongue with yellow fur.

DIRECTIONS

To be taken orally, 9g each time, twice a day

PRECAUTION

Don't angry, and don't eat sharp flavors, Contraindicated in cold of insufficiency type.

149 DANZHI XIAOYAO WAN（丹栀逍遥丸）

Ease Pill Added with Moutan Bark and Capejasmine Fruit

PRINCIPAL INGREDIENTS

Moutan bark (Cortex Moutan Radicis), Capejasmine fruit (Fructus Gardeniae), Bu-

pleurum root (Radix Bupleuri), Chinese angelica root (Radix Paeoniae), White peony
root (Radix Paeoniae Alba), Tuckahoe (Poria), Bighead atractylodes rhizome (Rhizoma Atractylodis Macrocephalae), Roasted
ginger (Rhizoma Zingiberis Recens Praeparata), Peppermint (Herba Menthae), Prepared licorice root (Radix Glycyrrhizae,
Praeparata)

FUNCTIONS

Soothing the liver, strengthening the spleen
and nourishing menstruation by regulating
the flow of blood.

INDICATIONS

Fire-transmission due to blood-deficiency of
the liver and spleen marked by irritability ,
or spontaneous perspiration of night sweat
or headache and xeroma, or irregular menstruation, pain and distension in the lower
abdomen, difficulty and pain in micturition.

DIRECTIONS

To be taken orally $1 \sim 2$ pills each time,
twice a day.

PRECAUTION

The recipe is contraindicated in patients
with frequent urination, enuresis, spontaneous emission due to fire-hyperactivity or

affection of damp-heat in the lower warmer.

150 SINI SAN（四逆散）

Powder for Treating Cold Limbs

PRINCIPAL INGREDIENTS

Bupleurum root（Radix Bupleuri）, White peony root（Radix Paeoniae Alba）, Fruit of immature citron or trifoliate orange（Fructus Aurantii Immaturus）, Prepared licorice root（Radix Glycyrrhizae Praeparata）

FUNCTIONS

Dispersing pathogens and alleviating mental depression, soothing the liver and regulating the spleen.

INDICATIONS

Patients with chronic hepatitis, cholecystitis, cholelithiasis, pancreatitis, neuralgia intercostalis and gastroneurosis marked by the symptoms of stagnation of the liver-Qi and the accumulation of the spleen- Qi and the accumulation of the spleen-Qi can be treated by the recipe.

DIRECTIONS

All the drugs listed above are to be decocted in water for oral administration 2～3g each time, two times a day.

PRECAUTION

Since it is indicated for cold limbs due to excess of heat which is caused by stagnation of Yang-Qi, the recipe is contraindicated in patients with cold limbs of other types.

151 SHUGAN WAN (舒肝丸)

Liver-soothing Bolus

PRINCIPAL INGREDIENTS

Sichuan chinaberry (Fructus Meliae Toosendan). Corydalis tuber (Rhizoma Corydalis). White peony root (Radix Paeoniae Alba). Turmeria (Rhizome Curcumae Longae). Auchlandia root (Radix Aucklandiae). Eagle wood (Lignum Aquilariae Resinatum). Round cardamon fruit (Fructus Amomi Rotundus). Amomum fruit (Fructus Amomi). Magnolia bark (Cortex Magnoliae Officinalis). Tangerine peel (Pericarpium Citri Reticulatae). Bitter orange (Fructus Aurantii). Poria (Poria)

FUNCTIONS

Regulating the liver, normalizing the function of the stomach and regulating the flow of Qi to alleviate pain.

INDICATIONS

Stagnation of the liver-Qi, manifested as distention and fullness in the hypochondria, poor appetite, dyspepsia, epigastralgia, epigastric upset, vomiting, belching and pantothen. Also advisable for hepatitis, gastritis, gastro-duodenal ulcer and hysteria due to stagnation of the liver-Qi.

DIRECTIONS

To be taken orally, 1 bolus each time, 2~3 times a day.

PRECAUTION

It should be used with great care for patients in pregnancy.

152 CHAIHU SHUGAN WAN（柴胡舒肝丸）

Bupleurum Pill for Relieving Liver-Qi

PRINCIPAL INGREDIENTS

Bupleurum root (Radix Bupleuri), Cyperus tuber (Rhizoma Cyperi), Tangerine Peel (Pericarpium Citri Reticulatae), Bitter orange (Fructus Aurantii), Chuanxiong rhizome (Rhizoma Ligustici Chuanxiong), White peony root (Radix Paeonia Alba), Prepared licorice (Radix Glycyrrhizae Praeparata)

FUNCTIONS

Soothing the liver and regulating the circulation of Qi. Promoting blood flow and nourishing the liver.

INDICATIONS

Chronic hepatitis, cholecystitis, chronic gastritis, gastroduodenal ulcer, gastric neurosis, hyperplasia of mammary glands, etc. Due to stagnation of the liver-Qi with the signs of hypochondriac pain, eructation, constipation, purplish red tongue, thin and whitish fur, taut and uneven pulse.

DIRECTIONS

To be taken orally, 6~9g each time, three times a day.

PRECAUTION

It is no longer used if the red tongue with little fur, dryness in mouth and pharynx occurred.

153 YUE JU WAN （越鞠丸）

Pill for Relieving Stagnancy

PRINCIPAL INGREDIENTS

Nutgrass flatsedge rhizome (Rhizoma Cyperi), Chuanxiong rhizome （Rhizoma Ligustici Chuanxiong）, Atractylodes rhizome (Rhizoma Atractylodis), Capejasmine fruit (Fructus Gardeniae), Medicated leaven (Massa Fermentata Medicinalis)

FUNCTIONS

Promoting the circulation of Qi to relieve

the stagnation.

INDICATIONS

Gastrointestinal neurosis, gastroduodenal ulcer, chronic gastritis, infectious hepatitis, cholecystitis, cholelithiasis, intercostal neuralgia, dysmenorrhea and others marked by symptoms of six kinds of stagnations can be treated by recipe.

DIRECTIONS

To be taken orally. 1 ~ 2 pills each time twice a day.

PRECAUTION

This recipe is indicated only for the stagnancies belonging to excess syndromes, stagnancies associated with deficiency type should not be treated only with this recipe.

154 SHUGAN ZHITONG WAN (舒肝止痛丸)

Tablet for Soothing the Liver to Alleviate Pain

PRINCIPAL INGREDIENTS

Bupleurum root (Radix Bupleuri), Scutellaria root (Radix Scutellariae), Chinese angelica root (Radix Angelicae Sinensis), White peony root (Radix Paeonia Alba), Curcuma root (Radix Curcumae), Aucklandia root (Radix Aucklandiae), Toosendan fruit (Fructus Meliae Toosendan), Chuanxiong rhizome (Rhizoma Ligustici Chuanxiong), Radish seed (Semen Raphani), Corydalis tuber (Rhizoma Corydalis), Bighead atractylodes rhizome (Rhizoma Atracty Lodis Macro-cephalae), Pinellia tuber (Rhizoma Pinelliae), Liquorice root (Radix Glycyrrhizae)

FUNCTIONS

Soothing the liver to regulating the flow of Qi, and promoting blood circulation to stop pain.

INDICATIONS

Neurosis, nonicterohepatitis, chronic gastritis, Syndrome of stagnation of the liver-Qi with the symptoms of fullness in the chest and hypochondrium, stomachache, eructation, acid regurgitation, mental oppression, and taut pulse.

DIRECTIONS

To be taken orally, 4~5g each time, twice a day.

155 ZUOJIN WAN (左金丸)

Liver-fire-purping and Stomach-Regulating Pill

PRINCIPAL INGREDIENTS

Coptis root (Rhizoma Coptidis), Evodia
fruit (Fructus Evodiae)

FUNCTIONS

purging Liver-fire, dispersing the depressed
liver-Qi, regulating the stomach-Qi and alleviating pain.

INDICATIONS

Dominant Liver-fire, attacking the stomach, manifested as pain in the hypochondriac, region, bitter taste, gastric upset, vomiting and acid regurgitation, dislike of hot
drinking

DIRECTIONS

To be taken orally, 3～6g each time, twice
a day.

PRECAUTION

Constant and long-term administration of it
is not advisable Great care should be taken
when exhibiting the drugs for those whose
spleen stomach functions are weak, other-
wise the stomach-Qi might be easily hurt.

156 WU JI WAN (戊己丸)

Liver-fire-purging and Spleen-stomach-
regulating Pill

PRINCIPAL INGREDIENTS

Coptis root (Rhizoma coptidis), Evodia fruit

(Fructus Evodiae), White peony root
(Radix Paeoniae Alba)

FUNCTIONS

Purging Liver-fire, regulating the functions
of the spleen and stomach.

INDICATIONS

Incoordination between the liver and the
stomach, marked by bitter taste, gastric
upset, vomiting and acid regurgitation, abdominal pain and dysentery.

DIRECTIONS

To be taken orally, 3~6g each time, twice
a day.

PRECAUTION ·

Never administered to avoid hot and stimulating food during taking it.

157 PING AN WAN (平安丸)

Bolus for Peaceful

PRINCIPAL INGREDIENTS

Cloves (Flos Caryophylli), Tangerine peel
(Pericarpium Citri Reticulate), Medicated
leaven massa (Fermentata Medicinalis),
Immature bitter orange (Fructus Aurantii),
Aucklandia root (Radix Aucklandiae),
Corydalis tuber (Rhizoma Corydalis), Areca
Seed (Semen Arecae), Apple (Apple),

Hawthorn fruit (Fructus Crataegi), Round cardamon seed (Semen Amomi Cardamomi)

FUNCTIONS

Regulating the flow of Qi and the stomach to alleviating pain.

INDICATIONS

Chronic hepatitis, chronic gastritis. The symptoms are distending pain in stomach, connected with the chest and hypochondrium, eructation, acid regurgitation, distress in the stomach, vexation, thin and yellow fur, taut pulse.

DIRECTIONS

To be taken orally, 1 bolus each time, twice a day.

PRECAUTION

Don't eat raw, cold and fat food.

158 XIANGSHA LIUJUNZI WAN (香砂六君子丸)

Pill of Costus and Amomum with Six Noble Ingredients

PRINCIPAL INGREDIENTS

Pilose asiabell root (Radix Dodonopsis pilosulae), Bighead atractylodes rhizome (Rhizome Atractylodis Macrocephalae), Poria (poria), Liquoric (Radix Glycyrrhizae),

Tangerine peel (Pericarpium Citri Reticulatae), Pinellia tuber (Rhizoma Pinelliae), Costus root (Radix Aucklandiae), Amomum fruit (Fructus Amomi)

FUNCTIONS

Supplementing Qi, invigorating the spleen and regulating the stomach.

INDICATIONS

Deficiency of the spleen and stomach with phlegm dampness and stagnation of Qi, marked by indigestion. eructation. anorexia. abdominal distension and fullness. loose stool. it may be used to treat peptic ulcer. chronic gastritis. disorder of stomach function. tion. etc.

DIRECTIONS

To be taken orally, 6~9g each time, 2~3 times a day.

PRECAUTION

The recipe should be administered with great care or not at all administered to those with high fever, or hyperactivity of fire due to Yin deficiency, or fullness due to stagnated Qi, or insufficiency of body fluid, or constipation.

159 JIUQI NIANTONG WAN（九气拈痛丸）

Nine-Qi Pill for Alleviating Pain

PRINCIPAL INGREDIENTS

Cyperus tuber (Rhizoma Cyperi), Galangal rhizome (Rhizoma Alpiniae Officinari), Tangerine peel (Pericarpium Citri Reticulatae), Curcuma root (Radix Curcumae), Zedoary (Rhizoma Zedoariae),Corydalis tuber (Rhizoma Corydalis), Areca seed (Semen Arecae), Trogopterus dung (Facces Trogopterorum)

FUNCTIONS

Regulating the flow of Qi and dispelling pathogenic cold. Promoting blood circulation to stop pain.

INDICATIONS

Acute or chronic gastritis, gastric neurosis, gastroduodenal ulcer, gastrectasia, gastricism, chronic diarrhea, coronary heart disease. Due to syndrome of accumulation of cold, stagnancy of the flow of Qi and Xue with the symptom of gastralgia, fullness in the chest and hypochondrium, anorexia, eructation, acid regurgitation.

DIRECTIONS

To be taken orally, 6g each time twice a day.

PRECAUTION

Don't eat raw, cold and fat food. Contraindication in pregnancy.

160 HUIXIANG JUHE WAN（茴香橘核丸）

Fennel Fruit and Tangerine Seed Pill

PRINCIPAL INGREDIENTS

Fennel fruit (Fructus Foeniculi), Tangerine seed (Semen Citri Reticulatae), Cassia Bark (Cortax Cinnamomi), Long pepper (Fructus Piper is Longi), Evodia fruit (Fructus Evodiae), Londera root (Radix Linderae), Aucklandia root (Radix Aucklandiae), Corydalis tuber (Rhizoma Corydalis), Toosendan fruit (Fructus Meliae Toosendan), Magnolia bark (Cortex Magnoliae Officinalis), Peach seed (Semen Persicae), Japanese sea tangle (Thellus Laminariae seu Eckloniae), Caulis Clematidis Armandii)

FUNCTIONS

Dispelling cold to alleviating pain. Soothing the liver and resolving masses.

INDICATIONS

Orchitis, epididymitis, hydrocele testis, herniation of intestine. The symptoms are scrotum swell, hard and pain, whitish tongue with white fur, taut or deep and tense pulse.

DIRECTIONS

To be taken orally, 1 bag each time twice a day.

PRECAUTION

Surgical therapy must be coordinated if the scrotum fester.

161 SUZI JIANGQI WAN（苏子降气丸）

Chaenomeles Fruit Pill

PRINCIPAL INGREDIENTS

Perilla fruit (Fructus Perillae), Magnolia bark (Cortex Magnoliae Officinalis), Peucedanum root (Radix Peucedani), Liquorice (Radix Glycyrrhizae), Prepared pinellia tuber (Rhizoma Pinelliae Praeparatum), Tangerine peel (Pericarpium citri Reticulatae), Eagle wood (Lignum Aquilariae Resinatum), Fresh ginger (Rhizoma Zingiberis Recens), Chinese angelica root (Radix Angelicae Sinensis), Chinese-date (Fructus Ziziphi Jujubae)

FUNCTIONS

Sending down the abnormally ascending Qi and resolving phlegm, warming the kidney and improving inspiration.

INDICATIONS

Reversed flow of Qi with accumulation of

phlegm, manifested as cough, dyspnea, feeling of fullness in the chest.

DIRECTIONS

To be taken orally, 6g each time. 1 ~ 2 times a day.

PRECAUTION

Not to be administered to patients with reddened tongue without coating due to Yin-deficiency.

162 YUE JU ER CHEN WAN (越鞠二陈丸)

Pill of Two Old Medicine for Relieving Stagnancy

PRINCIPAL INGREDIENTS

Nutgrass flatsedge rhizome (Rhizoma Lyperi), Atractylodes rhizome (Rhizoma Atractylodis), Tangerine peel (Pericarpium citri Reticulatae), Poria (Poria), Chuanxiong rhizome (Rhizoma Ligustici Chuanxiong), Medicated leaven (Massa Fermentata Medicinalis), Germinated barley (Fructus Hordei Germinatus), Liguorice (Radix Glycyrrhizae), Pinellia tuber (pinellia ternata)

FUNCTIONS

Invigorating the spleen to promote digest, promoting circulation of Qi to relieve melancholia, eliminating dampness and phlegm.

INDICATIONS

Choking and stuffiness Sensation in chest and diaphragm, nausea and.

DIRECTIONS

To be taker orally, two or three times a day with one bolus each time.

PRECAUTION

Contraindicated in patients with deficiency of Qi and Yang.

163   KUAN XIONG QI WU JI （宽胸气雾剂）

Aerosol for Soothing the Chest Oppression

PRINCIPAL INGREDIENTS

Borneol (Borneolum), Asarum herb oil （细辛油）, Sandalwood oil （檀香油）, Galangal rhizome oil （高良姜油）, Long pepper oil （荜拔油）

FUNCTIONS

Dissipating pathogenic cold, promoting circulation of Qi and blood, inducing resuscitation.

INDICATIONS

Syndrome of inhabitation of chest Yang and obstruction of heart-vessels by pathogenic cold with signs of chest pain radiating to the back or vice versa, cyanotic lips and extremities, shortness of breath, asthma,

white and greasy coating of tongue, deep
and slow pulse.

DIRECTIONS

Taken at the onset of angina pectoris, spray
inhaling by mouth.

PRECAUTION

Avoid angry and invasion by mouth.

I -11   Prescriptions for Treating Blood Disorder
理血剂

164   HEYE WAN（荷叶丸）

Bolus of Lotus Leaf

PRINCIPAL INGREDIENTS

Lotus leaf (Folium Nelumbinis), Japanese
thistle (Herba seu Radix cirsii Japonici),
Field thistle (Herba Cephalanoploris),
Scutellaria root (Radix Scutellariae), Dried
rehmannia root (Radix Rehmanniae), Co-
gongrass rhizome (Rhizoma Imperannia),
Scrophularia root (Radix Scrophulariae),
White peony root (Radix Paeoniae Alba),
Chinese angelica root (Radix Angelicae
Sinensis)

FUNCTIONS

Eliminating pathogenic heat from the

blood, removing blood stasis and arresting
bleeding.

INDICATIONS

Bleeding due to blood-heat, such as epistaxis, hemoptysis, hematemesis hematuria,
hemafecia, metrorrhagia and metrostaxis.

DIRECTIONS

To be taken orally, two or three times a day
with one bolus each time.

PRECAUTION

Contraindicated in bleeding due to deficiency of Qi.

165 BAIBU ZENGLI WAN （百补增力丸）

Bolus for Restorating Physical Strength

PRINCIPAL INGREDIENTS

Medicated leaven （Massa Fermentata Med-
icinalis）, Tangerine peel （Pericarpium Citri
Reticulatae）, White peony root （Radix
Paeoniae Alba）, Germinated barley （Fruc-
tus Hordei Germinatus）, Atractylodes rhizome （Rhizoma Atractylodis）, Rice sprout
（Fructus Oryzae Germinatus）, Hawthorn
fruit （Fructus Crataegi）, Chuangxiong rhizome （Rhizoma Ligustici Chuangxiong）,
Magnolia bark （Cortex Magnoliae Offici-
nalis）, Nutgrass flatsedge rhizome （Rhi-

zoma Cyperi), Ginseng (Radix Ginseng),
Rhubarb (Radix et Rhizoma Rhei), Chinese
yam (Rhizoma Dioscoreae), Prepared a-
conite root (Radix Aconiti Praeparata), Lo-
tus leaf (Folium Nelumbinis), Japanese
thistle (Herba Seu Radix cirsii Japonici),
Field thistle (Herba Cephalanoploris), Co-
gongrass rhizome (Rhizoma Imperatae),
Moutan bark (Cortex Moutan Radicis),
Bighead atractylodes rhizome (Rhizoma A-
tractylodis Macrocephalae), Rubia root
(Radix Rubiae), Astragalus root (Radix
Astragli Seu Hedysari), Pilose asiabell root
(Radix Codonopsis Pilosulae)

FUNCTIONS

Supplementing Qi, nourishing blood and arresting bleeding.

INDICATIONS

All kind of chronic hemarrhagia or hemator-
rhea with signs of weariness fatigue, shortness of breath, dizzying poor appetite.

DIRECTIONS

To be taken orally, twice a day with 1 or 2
bolus each time.

PRECAUTION

Avoid overworking and angry.

166 HUAIJIAO WAN (槐角丸)

Pill of Sophora Fruit

PRINCIPAL INGREDIENTS

Sophora fruit (Fructus Sophorae), Sanguisorba root (Radix Sanguisorbae), Ledebouriella root (Radix Ledebouriellae), Scutellaria root (Radix Scutellariae), Chinese angelica root (Radix Angelicae Sinensis)

FUNCTIONS

Cooling blood, stopping bleeding, eliminating dampness and toxic material.

INDICATIONS

It is indicated for cases with hematochezia or bleeding from the hemorrhoids. But its blood-cooling and hemostatic effect is stronger than the above prescription and is more suitable for those with severe retention of dampness-heat.

DIRECTIONS

To be taken orally, 6~9g each times, 1~2 times a day.

PRECAUTION

It is not advisable for the pregnancy women.

167 XIJIAO DIHUANG WAN (犀角地黄丸)

Pill of Cornu Rhinocerotis and Rehmanniae

PRINCIPAL INGREDIENTS

Dried rehmannie root (Radix Rehmanniae),
Moutan bark (Cortex Moutan Radicis),
Red peony root (Radix Paeoniae Rubra),
Rhinoceros horn (Cornu Rhinocerotis)

FUNCTIONS

Clearing away the heat evil in yingfen, cooling the blood, dispersing blood stasis and stopping bleeding.

INDICATIONS

Mainly for cases of hematemesis, epistaxis, hematuria, hemafecia, or skin rashes of dark purplish color, with rough and prickly fur on the tongue and rapid pulse, which are resulting from the extravasation of blood in case of the heat evil entering xuefen.

DIRECTIONS

To be taken orally, 1 bag each time, 1~2 times a day

PRECAUTION

Contraindicated in patients with deficiency of Yin

168 FUFANG DANSHEN PIAN（复方丹参片）

Compound Tablet of Red Sage Root

PRINCIPAL INGREDIENTS

Red sage root (Radix Salviae Multiorrhizae). Notoginseng (Radix Notoginseng). Borneol (Borneolum)

FUNCTIONS

Promoting blood circulation, removing blood stasis, inducing resuscitation by means of aromatics and regulating the blood flow of Qi to alleviate pain.

INDICATIONS

Coronary heart disease, angina pectoris and oppressed feeling in the chest.

DIRECTIONS

To be taken orally, 3 tablets each time, 3 times a day.

PRECAUTION

It is contraindicated in pregnancy.

169 FUFANG DANSHEN ZHUSHEYE（复方丹参注射液）

Compound Injection of Red Sage Root

PRINCIPAL INGREDIENTS

Red sage root (Radix Salviae Miltiorrhizae). Dalbergia wood (Lignum Dalbergiae Odoriferae)

FUNCTIONS

Promoting blood circulation, removing

blood stasis and improving microcircu-
lation.

INDICATIONS

Coronary heart disease and angina pectoris.

DIRECTIONS

Intramuscular injection, 2～4ml each time,
1～4 times a day. Intravenous injection,
4ml each time, once a day, it can only be
used after being diluted with 20ml of 50%
glucose injection. Intravenous drip, 10～
16ml once a day, it can only be used after
being diluted with 100～150ml of 50% glucose injection.

PRECAUTION

It is contraindicated in pregnancy.

170 XUEFU ZHUYU WAN (血府逐瘀丸)

Pill for Removing Blood Stasis in the Chest

PRINCIPAL INGREDIENTS

Chinese angelica root (Radix Angelicae
Sinensis), Chuanxiong rhizome (Rhizoma
Ligustici Chuanxiong), Red peony root
(Radix Paeoniae Rubra), Peach kernel (Se-
men Persicae), Safflower (Flos Carthami),
Achyranthes root (Radix Achyranthis
Bidentatae), Bupleurum root. (Radix Bu-
pleuri), Balloonflower root (Radix Platyco-

di）， Fruit of citron or trifoliate orange
(Fructus Aurantii)， Dried root of rehman-
nia （Radix Rehmanniae）， Licorice root
(Radix Glycyrrhizae）

FUNCTIONS

Promoting blood circulation to remove
blood stasis and promoting circulation of Qi
to relieve pain.

INDICATIONS

Coronary heart disease， cerebral thrombo-
sis， thromboangiitis obliterans， hyperten-
sion， cirrhosis of liver， dysmenorrhea，
amenia， postabortal retention of placenta，
headache， chest pain and hypochondriac
pain marked by stagnancy of Qi and blood
stasis can be treated by the recipe.

DIRECTIONS

To be taken orally two pill each time， twice
a day.

PRECAUTION

1. Since this recipe is mainly composed of
   drugs for removing blood stasis， it
   should not be used to treat the syndrome
   without distinct stasis.

2. It is contraindicated in pregnancy.

171 YUANHU ZHITONG PIAN（元胡止痛片）

Tablet of Corydalis Tuber for Alleviating
Pain

PRINCIPAL INGREDIENTS

Corydalis tubert (Rhizome Corydalis),
Bahurian angelica root （Radix Angelicae
Dahuricae）

FUNCTIONS

Promoting blood circulation to remove
blood stasis and regulating the flow of Qi to
alleviate pain.

INDICATIONS

Abdominalgia, stomachalgia, headache,
dysmenorrhea pain in the waist and lower
extremities, hepatalgia, etc.

DIRECTIONS

To be taken orally in case of pain, or 4～6
tablets each time, 2～3 times a day.

PRECAUTION

Patients who are very weak physically
should be treated with the recipe very carefully; it is contraindicated in pregnancy.

172 SHI XIAO SAN （失笑散）

Wonderful Powder for Relieving Blood
Stagnation

PRINCIPAL INGREDIENTS

Cat-tail pollen （Pollen Typhae）, Trogopterus dung (Faeces Trogopterorum)

FUNCTIONS

Promoting blood circulation by removing blood stasis, alleviating dysmenorrhea by adjusting menstruation.

INDICATIONS

Coronary disease, ectopic pregnancy, tumor, amenia, dysmenorrhea, persistant lochia after delivery, clinacteric syndrome etc., due to blood stagnation.

DIRECTIONS

To be taken orally, mixing with wine or decocting by wrapped with cloth, 6～9g each time, twice a day.

PRECAUTION

Contraindicated in syndrome of blood deficiency and syndrome without blood stagnation.

173 BIEJIA JIANWAN (鳖甲煎丸)

Pill of Fresh-Water Turtle Shell

PRINCIPAL INGREDIENTS

Fresh-water turtle shell (Carapax Trionycis), Bupleurum root (Radix Bupleuri), Cinnamom twig (Ramulus Cinnamomi), Pyrrosia Leaf (Folium Pyrrosiae), Magnolia bark (Cortex Magnoliae Officinalis),

Rhuberb (Radix et Rhizoma Rhei), Scutellaria root (Radix Scutellariae), Niter (Nitrum), Dried ginger (Rhizoma Zingiberis), Moutan bark (Cortex Moutan Radicis), Chinese trumpetcreeper (Flos Campsis), Pilose asiabell root (Radix codonopsis pilosulae)

FUNCTIONS

Softening masses, dispersing stagnation, removing blood stasis, activating blood circulation and eliminating phlegm.

INDICATIONS

It is indicated for cases of chronic malaria with splenomegaly, emaciation, diminish tongue, wiry and small pulse, which are attributive to deficiency of both vital energy and blood, and stagnation of phlegm and blood in the hypochondrium. The effect of removing blood stasis and activating blood circulation of this prescription is stronger than the above one.

DIRECTIONS

To be taken orally, 1~2 bolus each time, 1 ~2 times a day.

PRECAUTION

It is contraindicated in pregnancy.

174 XIAO SHUAN ZAI ZAO WAN（消栓再造丸）

Bolus for Removing Thrombus to Recover Functions

PRINCIPAL INGREDIENTS

Red sage root（Radix Salviae Miltiorrhizae）, Notoginseng（Radix Notoginseng）, Chuangxiong rhizome（Rhizoma Ligustici Chuangxiong）, Gastrodia tuber（Rhizoma Gastrodiae）, Storax（Styrax Liquidus）, Eagle Wood（Lignum Aguilariae Resinatum）, Ginseng（Radix Ginseng）

FUNCTIONS

Removing blood stasis and clearing blood vessels by promoting circulation of blood and Qi, inducing resuscitation.

INDICATIONS

Ischemic brain and heart disease in acute restoration and sequel stage.

DIRECTIONS

To be taken orally, twice a day with 1 or 2 bolus each time.

PRECAUTION

Avoid overworking and angry.

175 YU FENG NING XIN PIAN（愈风宁心片）

Tablet for Expelling Internal Wind to Relieve Mental Stress

PRINCIPAL INGREDIENTS

Pueraria root (Radix Puerariae)

FUNCTIONS

Anti-hypertension, promoting the circulation of blood of the heart and brain

INDICATIONS

Coronary disease, angina cordis, slight hypertension, meniere's disease, sudden deafness.

DIRECTIONS

To be taken orally, three times a day with 5
tablets each time.

PRECAUTION

Avoid overworking and angry.

176 DA HUANG ZHE CHONG WAN (大黃䗪虫丸)

Pill of Fibraurea Stem and Ground Beetle

PRINCIPAL INGREDIENTS

Ground beetle (Eupolyphagaseu Steleophaga), Leech (Hirudo), Peach Kernel (Semen
Persicae), Gradfly (Tabanus), Bitter apricot kernel (semen Armeniacae Amarum),
Scutellaria root (Radix Scutellariae), Pre-
Pared rhubarb (Radix et Rhizoma Rhei
praeparata), Dried rehmannia root (Radix

Rehmanniae), White peony root (Radix Paeoniae Alba), Liguorice (Radix Glycyrrhizae)

FUNCTIONS
Removing blood stasis and lumps clearing and activating the channels.

INDICATIONS
Hysteromyoma, tuberculosis of endometrium and fallopian tubes, chronic hepatitis, hepatocirrhosis etc, due to blood stasis and thus loss nourishing of body by blood and fluid.

DIRECTIONS
To be taken orally, three times a day with 3g each time.

PRECAUTION
Contraindicated in pregnant woman and amenia due to deficiency of blood.

177 GUANXIN ER HAO FANG (冠心 II 号方)
Recipe No. II for Coronary Heart Disease

PRINCIPAL INGREDIENTS
Chuanxiong rhizome (Rhizoma Ligustici Chuanxiong), Red sage root (Radix Salviae Miltiorrhizae), Safflower (Flos Carthami), Red Peony root (Radix Paeoniae Rubra), Dalbergia wood (Lignum Dalbergiae Odor-

iferae)

FUNCTIONS

Promoting blood circulation and removing blood stasis to relieve pain.

INDICATIONS

Coronary heart disease, angina pectoris, cardiac infarction or cerebral thrombosis or cerebral embolism in their initial stages can be treated by the recipe.

DIRECTIONS

To be taken orally 6 ~ 9g each time, 3 ~ 5 times a day.

PRECAUTION

Patients with menorrhagia and the deficiency of blood but without blood stasis should not be treated with this recipe. Pregnant women are especially forbidden to use the recipe in case abortion occurs.

178 JIOU XING DAN (救心丹)

Pill for Emergent Treating of Heart Disease

PRINCIPAL INGREDIENTS

Ginseng (Radix Ginseng), Cow-bezoare (Calculus Boris), Borneol (Borneolum), Musk (Moschus), Toad venom (Venenum Bufonis), Pearl, Notoginseng (Radix Notoginseng)

FUNCTIONS

Supplementing Qi to strengthen heart, promoting circulation of blood and Qi and arresting pain by removing blood stasis.

INDICATIONS

Heart pain, oppressive sensation in the chest, palpitation, shortness of breath, perspiration, pale tongue, thready pulse.

DIRECTIONS

To be taken sublingually or orally, twice a day with 1~2 pills each time.

PRECAUTION

If the pain relieved no longer use. It shouldn't be used for long and contraindicated in pregnant women.

I-12 Prescriptions for Tonifying
补益剂

179 SI JUNZI WAN (四君子丸)
Pill of Four Noble Drugs

PRINCIPAL INGREDIENTS

Ginseng (Radix Ginseng), Bighead atra Poria (Poria), Prepared licorice root (Radix Glycyrrhizae Praeparata)

FUNCTIONS

Replenishing Qi and strengthening the spleen.

INDICATIONS

The recipe can be modified to treat deficiency of Qi of the spleen and stomach as seen in cases of indigestion, chronic gastroenteritis, anemia, hypoproteinemia, chronic dysentery and various chronic disorders.

DIRECTIONS

To be taken orally, 5~7g each time, twice a day.

PRECAUTION

1. Prolonged administration of the recipe may lead to symptoms of dry mouth and tongue, thirst, restlessness and so on.

2. The recipe should be administered with great care or not at all administered to those with high fever, or hyperactivity of fire due to Yin deficiency, or fullness due to stagnated Qi, or insufficiency of body fluid, or excessive thirst and constipation.

180 WUJIASHEN CHONGJI (五加参冲剂)

Acanthopanax Infusion

PRINCIPAL INGREDIENTS

Pilose asiabell root (Radix Codonopsis Pilo-

sulae）, Ophiopogon root （Radix Ophio-
pogonis）, Wolfberry fruit （Fructus Lycii）

FUNCTIONS

Moistening the lung, promoting the production of body fluid, strengthening the spleen
and stomach and nourishing the liver and
kidney.

INDICATIONS

Weakness, dizziness, dimeyesight, soreness
in the waist, seminal emission, fatigue and
hypodynamia.

DIRECTIONS

To be taken orally after being infused in
boiling water, 10g each time, twice a day.

PRECAUTION

Since it has an astringent effect, it is neither fit for patients whose exopathogen has
not been dispelled, nor for those with hyperactivity of heat due to summer -heat diseases, but without impairment of Qi and
body fluid.

181 BUZHONG YIQI WAN （补中益气丸）

Bolus for Reenforcing Middle-Jiao and
Replenishing Qi

PRINCIPAL INGREDIENTS

Pilose asiabell root （Radix Codonopsis pilosulae), Astragalus root (Radix Astragali seu Hedysari), Liquorice (Radix Glycyrrhizae), Big-head atractylodes rhizome (Rhizoma Atractylodis, Macrocephalae), Chinese angelica root (Radix Angelicae Sinensis), Cimicifuga rhizome (Rhizoma Cimicifugae), Bupleurum root (Radix Bupleuri), Tangerine peel (Pericarpium Citri Reticulatae)

FUNCTIONS

Strengthening the Middle-jiao, replenishing Qi and elevating Yang to treat Prolapses of the internal organs.

INDICATIONS

Deficiency of the spleen and stomach and sinking of the Qi of middle-jiao, manifested as lassitude, poor appetite, abdominal distention, chronic diarrhea, proctoptosis and hysteroptosis.

DIRECTIONS

To be taken orally, 1 bolus each time, 2～3 times a day.

PRECAUTION

Patients with the impairment of body fluid and Qi after illness, it's better to prescribe this recipe together with other drugs.

182 LIUJUNZI WAN (六君子丸)

Pill of Six Ingredients

PRINCIPAL INGREDIENTS

Pilose asiabell root (Radix Codonopsis Pilosulae), Bighead atractylodes rhizome (Rhizoma Atractylodis Macrocephalae), Tangerine peel (Pericarpium Citri Reticulatae), Poria (Poria), Liguorice (Radix Glycyrrhizae), Prepared Pinellia tuber (Pinellia Ternata Preparat)

FUNCTIONS

Strengthening the spleen to supplement Qi, eliminating dampness and removing phlegm.

INDICATIONS

Chronic gastritis, chronic enteritis, chronic gastric and duodenal ulcer, chronic bronchitis etc., with signs of poor appetite dyspepsia, diarrhea or loose stool, weariness, oppressive sensation in the epigastrium after eating, sallow complexion, pallid tongue, slow feeble pulse, ect. that caused by accumulation of dampness and phlegm due to deficiency of Qi of the spleen of stomach.

DIRECTIONS

To be taken orally, two or three times a day with 6~9g each time.

PRECAUTION

Avoid eating cool, uncooked, pungent and greasy food.

183 SHENLING BAIZHU SAN (参苓白术散)

Powder of Ginseng, Poria and Bighead Atractylodes

PRINCIPAL INGREDIENTS

Lotus seed (Semen Nelumbinis), Job's-tears seed (Semen Coicis), Amomum fruit (Fructus Amomi), Platy codon root (Radix Platycodi), White hyaciath bean (Semen Dolichris Album), Poria (Poria), Ginseng (Radix Ginseng), Licorice root (Radix Glycyrrhizae), Bighead atractylodes rhizome (Rhizoma Atractylodis Macrocephalae), Chinese yam (Rhizoma Dioscoreae)

FUNCTIONS

Nourishing Qi and strengthening the spleen, regulating the stomach and eliminating dampness.

INDICATIONS

In addition, the recipe can be modified to deal with such cases as indigestion, chronic gastroenteritis anemia, nephrotic syndrome, chronic nephritis and other chronic disorders that are ascribable to stagnation of dampness due to deficiency of the spleen.

DIRECTIONS

To be taken orally，6～9g each time，three
times a day.

PRECAUTION

The recipe should be carefully administered
to patients with hyperactivity of fire due to
Yin deficiency; and should be used with dis-
cretion by patients associated with deficiency of both Qi and Yin，or deficiency of Yin
complicated with deficiency of the spleen.

184 JINGUI SHENQI WAN（金匮肾气丸）

Kidney-Qi-Tonifying Pill

PRINCIPAL INGREDIENTS

Prepared rehmannia root（Radix Rehmannia
Praeparata），Chinese Yam（Rhizoma Dios-
coreae），Dogwood fruit（Fructus Corni），
Poria（Poria），Oriental water plantain rhi-
zome（Rhizoma Alismatis），Moutan bark
（Cortex Moutan Radicis），Prepared aconite
root（Radix Aconiti Lateralis Praeparata），
Cinnamon bark（Cortex Cinnamomi）

FUNCTIONS

Tonifying the kidney-Qi and invigorating
the gate of life.

INDICATIONS

The deficiency of the kidney-Qi and decline of the fire from the gate of life, manifested as lassitude in the loins and legs, acute pain in the lower abdomen, cold lower limbs, polyuria in males due to diabetes and dysuria in females due to the pressure of fetus.

DIRECTIONS

To be taken orally, 8 pills each time, three times a day.

PRECAUTION

It is not advisable to administer this recipe for patients with hyperactivity of fire due to Yin deficiency and impairment of body fluid due to dryness-heat.

185 JISHEN SHENQI WAN (济生肾气丸)

Pill for Invigorating Kidney Energy

PRINCIPAL INGREDIENTS

Achyranthes root (Radix Achyranthis Bidentata), Plantain seed (Semen Planta-ginis), Bark of Chinese cassia tree (Cortex Cinnamomi), Prepared rehmannia root (Radix Rehmanniae), Chinese yam (Rhizome Dioscoreae), Dogwood fruit (Fructus Corni), Moutan bark (Cortex Moutan Radicis), Poria (Poria), Prepared aconite root (Radix Aconiti Praeparata)

FUNCTIONS

Warming and invigorating kidney-Yang,
and promoting diuresis.

INDICATIONS

Mainly for cases attributive to insufficiency
of kidney-Yang, manifested as lumbago,
flaccidity of legs, cold sensation over the
lower extremities oliguria or polyuria, cor-
pulent pale tongue, sunken and weak pulse.

DIRECTIONS

To be taken orally, 1～2 pills each times,
twice a day.

PRECAUTION

It is not advisable to administer this recipe
for patients with hyperactivity of fire due to
Yin deficiency.

186 YOUGUI WAN（右归丸）

Yougui Bolus

PRINCIPAL INGREDIENTS

Prepared rehmannia root (Radix Rehmanniae Praeparata), Dodder seed (Semen Cuscutae), Chinese angelica root (Radix Angelicae Sinensis), Chinese yam (Rhizome
Dioscoreae), Dogwood fruit (Fructus
Corni), Eucommia bark (Cortex Eucommi-

ae), Prepared aconite root (Radix Aconiti Praeparata), Bark of Chinese cassia tree (Cortex Cinnamomi)

FUNCTIONS

Warming and invigorating kidney-Yang.

INDICATIONS

Manifested as lumbago, cold limbs, shortness of breath, fatigue, impotence, nocturnal emission, pale tongue, small pulse, etc.

DIRECTIONS

To be taken orally, 1～2 pills each time, twice a day.

PRECAUTION

It is not advisable to administer this recipe for patients with hyperactivity of fire due to Yin deficiency and impairment of body fluid due to dryness-heat.

187   QUAN LU WAN (全鹿丸)

Pill of Deer's Embryo

PRINCIPAL INGREDIENTS

Deer's embryo, Cynomorium (Herba Cynomorii), Pilose asiabell root (Radix Codonopsis Pilosulae), Schisandra fruit (Fructus Schisandrae), Chinese yam (Rhizome Dioscoreae), Dried rehmannia root (Radix Rehmanniae), Prepared rehmannia root (Radix Rehmanniae Praeparata), Lucid asparagus root (Radix Asparagi), Psoralea fruit (Fructus Psoraleae), Achyranthes root (Radix Achyranthis Bidentatae), Dodder seed (Semen Cuscutae), Chuanxiong rhizome (Rhizome Ligustici Chuanxiong), Eagle wood (Lignum Aguilariae Resinatum)

FUNCTIONS

Replenishing the vital essence, tonifying the kidney -Yin and nourishing the bone marrow.

INDICATIONS

Marked by lassitude in the loins and legs, mental fatigue, dry mouth, night sweat, spermatorrhea, tinnitus and dim eyesight, metrorrhagia or metrostaxis, leukorrhagia.

DIRECTIONS

To be taken orally, 1 bolus each time twice a day.

PRECAUTION

Don't eat cold food. It is contraindicated in pregnancy.

188 GUILING JI (龟龄集)

Longevity Powder

PRINCIPAL INGREDIENTS

Ginseng (Radix Ginseng), Pilose antler
(Cornu Cervi pantotrichum), Sea horse
(Hippocampus), Desertliving cistanche
(Herba Cistanchis), Dodder seed (Semen
Cuscutae), Flatstem milkvetch seed (Se-
men Astragali Complanati), Psoralea fruit
(Fructus Psorale), Prepared aconite root
(Radix Aconiti Lateralis Praeparata),
Epimedium (Herba Epimedii)

FUNCTIONS

Nourishing the kidney, strengthening Yang
and replenishing the vital essence.

INDICATIONS

Symptoms caused by decline of fire from the
gate of life and deficiency of the kidney
essence, manifested as mental tiredness,
cold and pain in loins and abdomen, impotence and seminal emission, metrorrhagia
and metrostaxis, leukorrhagia and sterility.
It can be used to treat the above symptoms
resulting from neurosism, chronic nephritis
and menopausal syndrome in women.

DIRECTIONS

To be taken with yellow rice or millet wine
or warm boiled water, 6g each time, once
or twice a day.

PRECAUTION

It is not advisable to administer this recipe for patients with hyperactivity of five due to Yin deficiency and impairment of body fluid due to dryness-heat.

189 HUAN SHAO DAN （还少丹）

Pill for Restoring Yang

PRINCIPAL INGREDIENTS

Desertliving cistanche (Herba cistanchis), Wolfberry fruit (Fructus Lycii), Cyathula root (Radix Cyathulae), Schisandra fruit (Fructus Schisandrae), Chinese yam (Rhizome Dioscoreae), Prepared rehmannia root (Radix Rehmanniae Praeparata), Poria (Poria), Eucommia bark (Cortex Eucommiae), Dogwood fruit (Fructus Corni), Morinda root (Radix Morindae Officinalis)

FUNCTIONS

Warming and invigorating kidney-Yang, preserving essence and tranquilizing.

INDICATIONS

Mainly for cases attributive to declination of kidney -Yang, which manifest as impotence, nocturnal emission, lumbago, weakness of knee joints, frequent nocturnal urination, fatigue, dizziness, amnesia, poor appetite, pale tongue with white and smooth pulse, sunken and pulse.

DIRECTIONS

To be taken orally, 1 bolus each time, once a day.

PRECAUTION

It is not advisable to administer this recipe for patients with hyperactivity of fire due to Yin deficiency.

190 BAN LONG WAN（斑龙丸）

Banlong Pill

PRINCIPAL INGREDIENTS

Antler glue (Colla Cornus Cervi), Poria (Poria), Dodder seed (Semen Cuscutae), Prepared rehmannia root (Radix Rehmanniae Praeparata), Psoralea fruit (Fructus Psoraleae)

FUNCTIONS

Nourishing and invigorating the kidney-essence, preserving sperm and tranquilizing

INDICATIONS

Mainly for cases of nocturnal emission, impotence or premature ejaculation accompanied with lumbago, tinnitus, nocturia, dizziness, fatigue, pale complexion, pale tongue with white fur, sunken and small, weak pulse, which are attributive to the impairment of kidney essence and the weakness of kidney-energy.

DIRECTIONS

To be taken orally, 1 bolus each time, twice a day.

PRECAUTION

It is not advisable to administer this recipe for patients with hyperactivity of fire due to Yin deficiency.

191　JI XUE TEN GAO（鸡血藤膏）

Spatholobus Stem Paste

PRINCIPAL INGREDIENTS

Spatholobus stem （Caulis Spatholobi）, Fresh cyathula root （Radix Cyathulae）, Fresh dipsacus root （Radix Dipsaci）, Black soybean （Semen Sojae Nigrum）, Safflower （Flos Carthami）

FUNCTIONS

Enriching and activating blood to regulate menstruation.

INDICATIONS

Anemia, menstrual disorder or rheuma-toid arthritis etc., that pertain to the syndrome of deficiency and stasis of blood with symptoms of numbness in the hands and feet, weakness and soreness in the bones and tendons, sallow or pale complexion, dizziness and tinnitus, lumbago, troubled flexibility in limbs, palpitation, difficult sleepiness etc..

DIRECTIONS

To be taken orally after dissolved in water and equal wine, twice a day with 9～15g each time.

PRECAUTION

Contraindicated in syndrome of deficiency of the spleen with loose stool.

192　EJIAO BUXUE GAO (阿胶补血膏)

Donkey-Hde Gelatin Paste for Replenishing Blood

PRINCIPAL INGREDIENTS

Donkey-hide gelatin (Colla Corri Asini), Astragalus root (Radix Astragari Seu Hedysari), Pilos asiabell root (Radix Codonopsis Pilosulae), Wolfberry fruit (Fructus Lycii), Prepared rehmannia root (Radix Rehmanniae Praeparate)

FUNCTIONS

Reinforcing the spleen and nourishing the lung, replenishing blood and Yin.

INDICATIONS

Pulmonary tuberculosis, hypotension, anemia, menstruation disorder, amenia etc., that pertain to the syndrome of deficiency of bloodand Qi of the spleen and lung, with signs of shortness of breath, weariness, spontaneous and profuse sweating, anorexia, asthemia distention in the chest and abdomen, sallow complexion with pale colored lips, stool disorder, pale tongue and thready feeble pulse.

DIRECTIONS

To be taken orally, twice a day with 15~ 30g each time.

PRECAUTION

Contraindicated in dyspepsia with stasis and accumulation of residue inside, contra-indicated in cold.

193 TIANWANG BUXIN DAN （天王补心丹）

Cardiotonic Bolus

PRINCIPAL INGREDIENTS

Dried rehmannia root (Radix Rehmanniae), Scorphularia root (Radix Scrophulariae), Ophiopogon root (Radix Ophiopogonis), Red sage root (Radix Salviae Multiorrhizae), Chinese angelica root (Radix Angelicae Sinensis), Grassleaved sweetflag rhizome (Rhizoma Acori Craminei), Pilose

asiabell root (Radix Codonopsis Pilosulae),
Poria (Poria), Schisandra fruit (Fructus
Schisandrae), Polygala root (Radix Poly-
galae), Spring date seed (Semen Ziziphi
Spinosae), Liquorice (Radix Glycyrrhizae)

FUNCTIONS

Replenishing Yin and nourishing the blood,
supplementing the heart and tranquilizing
the mind.

INDICATIONS

The deficiency of the heart-Yin, marked
by palpitation, amnesia, insomnia, dreaminess, ulceration of the mouth and tongue,
and constipation.

DIRECTIONS

To be taken orally, 1 bolus each time,
twice a day.

PRECAUTION

As the recipe has the effects of moistening
dryness and relaxing the bowels, it is not
suitable for patients with weakness of gastrointestinal or with diarrhea.

194 LIU WEI DIHUANG WAN (六味地黄丸)

Pill of Six Ingredients with Rehmannia

PRINCIPAL INGREDIENTS

Prepared rehmannia root (Radix Rehmanniae Praeparata), Dogwood fruit (Fructus Corni), Moutan bark (Cortex Moutan Radicis), Chinese yam (Rhizoma Dioscoreae), Poria (Poria), Oriental water plentain (Rhizoma Alismatis), Rhizoma

FUNCTIONS
Nourishing the Yin of liver and kidney.

INDICATION
Deficiency of liver-Yin and kidney-Yin, and flaring-up of fire of deficiency type, manifested as lassitude in loins and knees, dizziness, vertigo, tinnitus, deafness, emission, night sweat, hectic, fever due to Yin-deficiency, red tongue with little fur, thready and rapid pulse.

DIRECTIONS
To be taken orally, 9g each time, twice a day.

PRECAUTION
Since it tends to be greasy lonics, the recipe should be administered carefully to patients with weakened function of the spleen in transporting and distributing nutrients and water.

195 QIJU DIHUANG WAN (杞菊地黄丸)
Pill of Wolfberry Fruit and Chrysanthe-

mum

PRINCIPAL INGREDIENTS

Wolfberry fruit (Fructus Lycii), Chrysanthemum flower (Flos Chrysanthemi), Prepared rehmannia root (Radix Rehmanniae Praeparata), Chinese yam (Rhizoma Dioscoreae), Dogwood fruit (Fructus Corni), Poria (Poria), Moutan bark (Cortex Moutan Radicis)

FUNCTIONS

Nourishing the liver and kidney refreshing the brain and improving eyesight.

INDICATIONS

Syndrome of deficiency of the liver and kidney Yin that characterized by vertigo, blurred vision, xerophthalmia and ophthalmagia, lacrimation when touch wind, photophobia, tinnitus or deafness, tidal fever, night sweating. It includes optic neuritis, retinitis, optic atrophy, chronic glaucoma, neurosism etc..

DIRECTIONS

To be taken orally, 9g each time, twice a day.

PRECAUTION

Avoid eating acid and cold food.

196　ZHI BAI DIHUANG WAN（知柏地黄丸）

Pill of Phellodendrom Bark and Moutan Bark

PRINCIPAL INGREDIENTS

Prepared rehmannia root (Radix Rehmanniae Praeparata), Dogwood fruit (Fructus Co-rni), Moutan bark (Cortex Moutan Radicis), Chinese Yam (Rhizoma Dioscoreae), Poria (Poria), Oriental water plantain (Rhizoma Alismatis), Phellodendrom bark (Cortex Phellodendri), Moutan bark (Coretex Moutan Radicis)

FUNCTIONS

Nourishing Yin and expelling pathogenic heat from the interior.

INDICATIONS

Latent heat in the interior of the body, manifested by fever at night and normal in the morning, absence of perspiration after fever subsides, polyphagia with emaciation, reddened tongue with little coating and rapid pulse.

The recipe can be modified for the treatment of pulmonary tuberculosis as well as other chronic consumptive diseases related to the above syndrome.

DIRECTIONS

To be taken orally, 1 ~ 2 boluses each times, three times a day.

PRECAUTION

The recipe has weak effect in reducing fever, but greater effect in nourishing Yin, therefore, it is not advisable for cases with severe fever and milder hectic Yin-deficiency.

197 QIWEI DUQI WAN（七味都气丸）

Pill of Seven Ingredients

PRINCIPAL INGREDIENTS

Prepared rehmannia root (Radix Rehmanniae Praeparata), Dogwood fruit (Fructus Corni), Chinese yam (Rhizoma Dioscoreae), Poria (Poria), Moutan bark (Cortex Moutan Radicis), Schisandra fruit (Fructus Schisandrae)

FUNCTIONS

Replenishing Yin to reduce pathogenic fire, nourishing the kidney and astringing the lung.

INDICATIONS

Syndrome of deficiency of the kidney Yin with signs of cough and asthmia, spontaneous emission, frequent micturition, weakness and soreness in loins and knees,

dizziness and tinnitus, dysphoria with feverish sensation, night sweating, red tongue
with little fluid, thready and rapid pulse.

DIRECTIONS

To be taken orally, 9g each time, three
times a day.

PRECAUTION

Contraindicated in cough and asthmia due to
excess syndrome, and emission and frequent
micturition due to deficiency of kidney
Yang.

198 ZUOGUI WAN（左归丸）

Kidney-Yin-Tonifying Bolus

PRINCIPAL INGREDIENTS

Prepared rehmannia root (Radix Rehmanniae Praeparata), Wolfberry fruit (Fructus
Lycii), Antler glue (Colla Crnus Cervi),
Glue of tortoise Plastron (Colla Plastri Testudinis), Dodder seed (Semen Cussutae),
Dogwood fruit (Fructus Corni), Chinese
yam (Rhizoma Dioscoreae), Achyranthes
root (Radix Achyranthis Bidentatae)

FUNCTIONS

Replenishing the vital essence, tonifying the
kidney -Yin and nourishing the bone marrow.

INDICATIONS

Symptoms due to deficiency of the kidney-Yin, marked by lassitude in the loins and legs, mental fatigue, dry mouth, night sweat, spermatorrhea, frequent fever of deficiency type, tinnitus and dim eyesight.

DIRECTIONS

To be taken orally before meals, 9g each time, twice a day.

PRECAUTION

Prolonged administration of the recipe is liable to obstruct the function of the spleen and stomach, for this reason, it is advisable to add into the recipe tangerine peel, amomum fruit or other drugs so as to regulate the flow of Qi to enliven the spleen and to avoid any disturbance with tonification.

199 DA BUYIN WAN (大补阴丸)

Bolus for Replenishing Vital Essence

PRINCIPAL INGREDIENTS

Phellodendron bark (Cortex Phellodendri), Wind-weed rhizome (Rhizoma Anemarrhenae), Prepared rhizome of rehmannia (Rhizoma Rehmanniae Praeparata), Tortoise plastron (Plastrum Testudinis)

FUNCTIONS

Nourishing Yin and purging pathogenic fire.

INDICATIONS

Equally, the above syndrome seen in cases of hyperthyroidism, renal tuberculosis, bone tuberculosis and diabetes can respond well to the treatment with the modified recipe.

DIRECTIONS

To be taken orally, 1 pill each time, twice a day.

PRECAUTION

The recipe is not advisable for patients with watery stool after meal.

200   ERZHI WAN (二至丸)

Erzhi Pill

PRINCIPAL INGREDIENTS

Eclipta (Herba Ecliptae), Glossy privet fruit (Fructus Ligustri Lucidi)

FUNCTIONS

Benefiting the liver and kidney and invigorating the Yin-blood.

INDICATIONS

Indicated for cases attributive to deficiency of the liver-Yin and kidney-Yin, manifested as insomnia, dreaminess, nocturnal emission, fatigue, dizziness, etc..

DIRECTIONS

To be taken orally, 1~2 boluses each time, twice a day.

PRECAUTION

It is better not to be administered for those with sputum and stagnation of body fluid.

201 ERDONG GAO （二冬膏）

Paste of Asparagus Root and Ophiopogen Root

PRINCIPAL INGREDIENTS

Lucid Asparagus root （Radix Asparagi）, Ophiopogen root （Radix Ophiopogonis）, Honey （Mel）

FUNCTIONS

Nourishing Yin to reduce pathogenic heat, tonifying the lung to arrest cough.

INDICATIONS

Syndrome of deficiency of Yin of the lung and kidney with signs of irritating dry cough with blood streak or hemoptysis, shortness of breath with oppressive sensation in chest, dryness in mouth, with desire of drinking, sore but not swelled celostomia, crimson tongue with little fur.

DIRECTIONS

To be taken orally, 9~15g each time, twice a day.

PRECAUTION

It is contraindicated in the syndrome of dampness-heat with phlegm.

202 SHOUWU WAN（首乌丸）

Pill of Fleece-Flower Root

PRINCIPAL INGREDIENTS

Fleece-flower root （Radix Polygoni Multiflori）, Dried rehmannia root （Radix Rehmannia）, Mulberry （Fructus Mori）, Glossy Privet fruit （Fructus Ligustri Lucidi）, Eclipta （Herba Ecliptae）, Sesame seed （Semen Sesami）, Dodder seed （Semen Cuscutae）, Achyranthes root （Radix Achyranthis Bidentatae）, Psoralea fruit （Fructus Psoraleae）, Honeysuckle flower （Flos Lonicerae）, Cherokee rose-hip （Fructus Rosae Laevigatae）

FUNCTIONS

Replenishing the liver and kidney essence to blackening hair.

INDICATIONS

The syndrome of deficiency of vital of the liver and kidney with signs of: haggard face, zygomatic flushing, dysphasia with a feverish sensation in the chest, palms, and soles, night sweating, dizzying, weakness and soreness in the knees and loins, spontaneous emission for man or scanty menstruation for woman, red tongue with little fluid and fur, deep and rapid pulse.

DIRECTIONS

To be taken orally, 6g each time, twice a day.

PRECAUTION

It is contraindicated in the syndrome of deficiency of Qi and Yang of the spleen and stomach. Avoid eating pungent food.

203 SHANSHEN GAO（桑椹膏）

Mulberry Paste

PRINCIPAL INGREDIENTS

Mulberry (Fructus Mori), Can Sugar （蔗糖）, Tartric acid （酒石酸）

FUNCTIONS

Replenishing the kidney and liver, nourishing blood, tranquilization, enriching body fluid and quenching thirst.

INDICATIONS

Vertigo, insomnia and amnesia, tinnitus, dryness in the mouth and throat, weakness and soreness in the loins, disphoria with feverish sensation in the chest, palms, and soles, zygomatic flushing and night sweating, spontaneous emission, constipation, thready and rapid pulse etc., due to deficiency of Yin of the liver and kidney, insuffticiency of body fluid and dryness of blood.

DIRECTIONS

To be taken orally, 15 ~ 30g each time, twice a day.

PRECAUTION

It is contraindicated in diarrhea due to invasion of asthemia spleen and stomach by pathogenic cold.

204 YUQUAN WAN (玉泉丸)

Diabetes Pill

PRINCIPAL INGREDIENTS

Pueraria root (Radix Puerariae), Snakegourd root (Radix Trichosanthis), Dried root of rehmannia (Radix Rehmanniae), Ophiopogon root (Radix Ophiopogonis)

FUNCTIONS

Promoting the production of body fluid to relieve thirst, clearing away heat to arrest irritability, and nourishing Yin and the kidney.

INDICATIONS

Diabetes.

DIRECTIONS

To be taken orally, 6g each time, 4 times a day, one course of treatment covers a month.

PRECAUTION

Since it tends to be greasy tonics, the recipe should be administered carefully to patients with weakened function of the spleen in transporting and distributing nutrients and water.

205 SANCAI FENGSHUI DAN (三才封髓丹)

Pill for Promoting Curing

PRINCIPAL INGREDIENTS

Prepared rehmannia root (Radix Rehmannia Praeparata), Lucid asparagus root (Radix Asparagi), Pilose asiabell root (Radix Codonopsis Pilosulae), Phellodendron bark (Cortex Phellodendri), Amomum fruit (Fructus Amomi), Desertliving Cistanche (Herba Cistanchis), Liguorice (Radix Glycyrrhizae)

FUNCTIONS

Nourishing Yin and reducing pathogenic fire supplementing Qi and promoting the production of body fluid.

INDICATIONS

Syndrome of deficiency of kidney Yin and hyperactivity of the ministrial fire with symptoms of seminal emission, premature ejaculation, dizziness, palpitation, disturbed sleep, tiredness, stomatocace red and dry tongue, rapid and thready pulse.

DIRECTIONS

To be taken orally, 9g each time, twice a day.

PRECAUTION

Don't eat acrid food.

206 JIAN BU WANG（健步丸）

Bolus for Vigorous Walking

PRINCIPAL INGREDIENTS

Phellodendron bark (Cortex Phellodendri), Prepared rehmannia root (Radix Rehmanniae Praeparata), Tortoise plastron (Plastrum Testudinis), Chinese angelica root (Radix Angelicae Sinensis), White peony root (Radix Paeoniae Alba), Cynomorium (Herba Cynomorii), Dried ginger (Rhizoma Zingi Beris), Tangerine peel (Pericarpium citri Reticulatae), Achyranthes root (Radix Achyranthis Bidentatae)

FUNCTIONS

Tonifying the liver and kidney, strengthening tendons and bones.

INDICATIONS

Artralgia-syndrome and flaccidity syndrome due to deficiency of essence of the liver and kidney, or sequel of poliomyelitis, myasthenia gravies, malnutrition, neuritis rheumatic arthritis.

DIRECTIONS

To be taken orally, one bolus each time, twice a day.

PRECAUTION

Don't eat acrid food

207　BAZHEN WAN（八珍丸）

Bolus of Eight Precious Ingredients

PRINCIPAL INGREDIENTS

Ginseng (Radix Ginseng), Bighead atractylodes rhizome (Rhizoma Atractylodis Macrocephalae), Poria (Poria), White Peony Root (Radix Paeoniae Alba), Chinese angelica root (Radix Angelicae Sinensis), Chuanxiong rhizome (Rhizoma Ligustici Huanxiong), Prepared rehmannia root (Radix Rehmanniae Praeparata), Prepared liguorice (Radix Glycyrrhizae Praeparata)

FUNCTIONS

Supplementing Qi and nourishing blood.

INDICATIONS

Anemia, chronic consumptive disease, chronic hepatitis, chronic cholecystitis gastrointestinal neurosis, insomnia , habitual abortion and carbunche etc. Pertain to deficiency of Qi and blood.

DIRECTIONS

To be taken orally, one bolus each time, twice a day.

PRECAUTION

It is contraindicated in excess syndrome with pathogenic heat. Don't overwork coitus and eat cold food.

208 SHIQUAN DABU WAN (十全大补丸)

Bolus of Ten Powerful Tonics

PRINCIPAL INGREDIENTS

Pilose asiabell root (Radix Codonopsis pilosulae), Bighead atractylodes rhizome (Rhizoma Atractylodis Macrocephalae), Poria (Poria), Liquorice (Radix Glycyrrhizae), Chinese angelica root (Radix Angelicae Sinensis), Chuanxiong rhizome (Rhizoma Ligustici Chuanxiong), White peony root (Radix Paeoniae Alba), Prepared rehman-

nia root (Radix Rehmanniae, Praeparata),
Astragalus root (Radix Astragali seu
Hedysari), Cinnamon bark (Cortex Cin-
namomi)

FUNCTIONS

Warming and nourishing Qi and blood.

INDICATIONS

Deficiency of both Qi and blood marked by
sallow complexion, short breath, palpitation, dizziness, spontaneous perspiration,
mental fatigue, lassitude of the extremities,
profuse menstruation, it also serves as a
supporting drug to detoxicating drugs in the
treatment of non-healing of ulcers due to
deficiency of Qi and blood.

DIRECTIONS

To be taken orally, 1 bolus each time, 2～3
times a day.

PRECAUTION

It is neither fit for patients whose exopathogen has not been dispelled, nor for
those with hyperactivity of heat due to summer-heat diseases, but without impairment
of Qi and body fluid.

209 DANGGUI BUXUE WAN（当归补血丸）
Pill of Chinese Angelica Root Invigorating

PRINCIPAL INGREDIENTS

Astragalus root (Radix Astragali seu Hedysari), Chinese angelica root (Radix Angelicae Sinensis)

FUNCTIONS

Invigorating vital energy and promoting blood production.

INDICATIONS

Mainly for cases of internal damage by over-strain, and deficiency of blood and vital energy, which are manifested as fever, restlessness, thirst, pulse bounding but weak on pressing.

DIRECTIONS

To be taken orally, 1 bolus each time 3 time a day.

PRECAUTION

The recipe should not be administered to those with heat-evil hidden interiorly and those with rapid pulse due to Yin deficiency.

210 SHENGMAI CHONGJI (生脉冲剂)

Infusion for Restoring Pulse Beating

PRINCIPAL INGREDIENTS

Dried rehmannia root (Radix Rehmanniae), Ophiopogon root (Radix Ophiopogonis), Schisandra fruit (Fructus Schisandrae)

FUNCTIONS

Supplementing vital energy, Promoting body fluid production, astringent Yin and stopping excessive perspiration.

INDICATIONS

Mainly for the cases with deficiency of both vital energy and Yin manifested as hyperhidrosis, shortness of breath, tiredness and small and weak pulse, and the cases of spontaneous perspiration and shortness of breath due to damage of the lung caused by chronic cough and damage of both vital energy and Yin.

DIRECTIONS

To be taken orally after being infused in boiling water, 10g each time, 2~3 times a day.

PRECAUTION

Since it has an astringent effect, it is neither fit for patients whose exopathogen has not been dispelled, nor for those with hyperactivity of heat due to summer -heat diseases, but without impairment of Qi and body fluid.

211 SHENMAI ZHUSHEYE（参麦注射液）

Injection of Ginseng and Ophiopogon Root

PRINCIPAL INGREDIENTS

Ginsheng (Radix Ginseng), Ophiopogon Root (Radix Ophiopogonis)

FUNCTIONS

Supplementing Qi, promoting the production of body fluid and curing prostration.

INDICATIONS

Syncope and Deficient syndrome characterized by dizzying, sweating palpitation, thirsty faint pulse, etc..

DIRECTIONS

Intramuscular or intravenous injection. Intramuscular: 2 ~ 4ml each time, twice a day. Intravenous: 5 ~ 10ml with 5% glucose injection 250ml by intravenous drip.

PRECAUTION

Don't used in the syndrome of deficiency of Yang and excess of Yin.

212 GUIPI WAN (归脾丸)

Ginseng Spleen-Invigorating Bolus

PRINCIPAL INGREDIENTS

Ginseng (Radix Ginseng), Chinese angelica root (Radix Angelicae Sinensis), Astragalus root (Radix Astragali seu Hedysari), Dried longan aril (Arillus Longan), Costus root (Radix Aucklandiae), Polygala root

(Radix Polygalae), Spying jujuba seed (Semen Ziziphi Spinosae), Liquoric (Radix Glycyrrhizae), Poria (Poria), Bighead atractylodes rhizome (Rhizoma Atractylodis Macrocephalae)

FUNCTIONS

Invigorating the spleen, nourishing the heart, replenishing Qi and enriching the blood.

INDICATIONS

Deficiency of Qi and blood due to dysfunction of the heart and spleen by palpitation, insomnia, anorexia, fatigue, and weakness, sallow, complexion, irregular menstruation, metrorrhagia and metrostaxis, leukorrhagia and aplastic anemia, and thrombocytopenic.

DIRECTIONS

To be taken orally, 1 bolus each time, 2~3 times a day.

PRECAUTION

The recipe should not be administered to those with heat-evil hidden interiorly and those with rapid pulse due to Yin deficiency.

213 RENSHEN JIANPI WAN (人参健脾丸)

Ginseng Spleen-Strengthening Bolus

PRINCIPAL INGREDIENTS

Ginseng (Radix Ginseng), Hawthorn fruit (Fructus Crataegi), Germinated barley (Fructus Hordei Germinatus), Medicated leaven (Massa Fermentata Medicinalis), Tangerine peel (Pericarpium citri Reticulatae), Bighead atractylodes rhizome (Rhizoma Atractylaodis Macrocephalae), Immature bitter orange (Fructus Aurantii Immaturus)

FUNCTIONS

Invigorating the spleen, regulating the flow of and promoting digestion.

INDICATIONS

Insufficiently of the spleen and stagnation of Qi, manifested as abdominal distention and poor appetite.

DIRECTIONS

To be taken orally, 1 bolus each times, 2 or 3 times a day.

PRECAUTION

The recipe should be carefully administered to patients with hyperactivity of fire due to Yin deficiency.

214 RENSHEN YANGRONG WAN (人参养荣

丸）

Ginseng Tonic Bolus

PRINCIPAL INGREDIENTS

Ginseng (Radix Ginseng), Astragalus root (Radix Astragli seu Hedysari), Bighead atractylodes rhizome (Rhizoma Atractylodis Macrocephalae), Poria (Poria), Prepared rehmannia root (Radix Rehmanniae Praeparata), Chinese angelica root (Radix Angelicae Sinensis), White peony root (Radix Paeoniae Alba), Cinnamon bark (Cortex Cinnamomi), Schisandra fruit (Fructus Schisandrae), Polygala root (Radix Polygalae), Tangerine peel (Pericarpium citri Reticulatae), Prepared liquorice (Radix Glycyrrhizae Praeparata)

FUNCTIONS

Invigorating and blood, tranquilizing mind and promoting mentality

INDICATIONS

For the treatment of mental fatigue and tiredness, poor appetite, loose stool, palpitation due to fright, ammesia, emaciation, spontaneous perspiration and night sweat, trichomadesis, and sallow complexion.

DIRECTIONS

To be taken orally, 1 bolus each time,

twice a day.

PRECAUTION

Patients with internal heat due to Yin deficiency is prohibited from taking this recipe, and for those with the impairment of body fluid and Qi after illness, it's better to prescribe this recipe together with other drugs.

215 RENSHEN GUBEN WAN (人参固本丸)

Ginseng Bolus for Strengthening Body's Essence

PRINCIPAL INGREDIENTS

Ginseng (Radix Ginseng), Chinese yam (Rhizoma Dioscorae), Dried rehmannia root (Radix Rehmannia), Prepared rehmannia root (Radix Rehmannia Praeparata), Ophiopogon root (Radix Ophiopogonis), Lucid asparagus root (Radix Asparagi), Poria (Poria), Dogwood fruit (Fructus Corni), Moutan bark (Cortex Moutan Radicis)

FUNCTIONS

Supplementing Qi and Ying. Reforcing body's basic materials and strengthening body's essence.

INDICATIONS

Consumptive disease, Tuberculosis, etc.

characterized by fatigue. Coughing hemoptysis, palpitation, dyspnea, soreness of waist, tinnitus, hectic fever and night sweating or constipation, dark urine and difficulty in micturition, red tongue with scanty fur, feeble, faint and rapid pulse.

DIRECTIONS

To be taken orally, one bolus each time, twice a day.

PRECAUTION

It is contradicted in cold.

216 RENSHEN LURONG WAN (人参鹿茸丸)

Ginseng and Pilose Antlfer Bolus

PRINCIPAL INGREDIENTS

Ginseng (Radix Ginseng), Pilose antler powder (Cornu Cervi Pantotrichum), Psoralea fruit (Fructus Psoraleae), Achyranthes root (Radix Achyranthis Bidentatae), Cordyceps (Cordyceps), Eucommia bark (Cortex Eucommiae), Longan aril (Arillus Longan), Dodder seed (Semen Cuscutae), Nutgrass flatsedge rhizome (Rhizoma Lyperi), Astragalus root (Radix Astragali Seu Hedysari), Morinda root (Radix Morindae Officinalis), Poria (Poria)

FUNCTIONS

Warming the kidney and strengthening Yang strengthening the spleen and replenishing Qi Nourishing the blood and enriching the primordial energy.

INDICATIONS

Consumptive disease, spontaneous emission, lumbago, irregular menstruation, gynecological disease etc. with symptoms of lassitude, cold extremities, blurred vision, tinnitus, spontaneous emission and night sweating, soreness in the waist and knee, delayed menarche, cold in uterus, mentrorrhagia and metrostaxis, laukorrhagia, pale tongue with white fur, feeble pulse.

DIRECTIONS

To be taken orally, one bolus each time, twice a day.

PRECAUTION

Avoid eating uncooked and cold food.

217 SHUYU WAN (薯蓣丸)

Pill of Chinese Yam

PRINCIPAL INGREDIENTS

Chinese yam (Rhizoma Dioscoreae), Rehmannia root (Radix Rehmanniae), White peony root (Radix Paeoniae Alba), Chinese angelica root (Radix Angelicae

Sinensis), Chuanxiong rhizome (Rhizoma Ligustici Chuanxiong), Bighead atractylodes rhizome (Rhizoma Atractylodis Macrocephalae), Donkey-hide gelatin (Colla Corii Asini), Ledebouriella root (Radix Ledebouriellae), Cinnamom twig (Ramulus Cinnamomi)

FUNCTIONS

Expelling wind and tonifying.

INDICATIONS

Mainly for consumptive diseases complicated by the attack of wind evil, manifested as dizziness, emaciation, fatigue, shortness of breath, spontaneous sweating alternate feeling of chills and fever, liability to catch cold, poor appetite, loose stools, sallow complexion, pale tongue with white fur, soft and weak pulse, which are attributive to deficiency of lung and spleen-energy, decrease of body resistance and impairment of healthy energy.

DIRECTIONS

To be taken orally, 5~10g each time, 2~3 times a day.

PRECAUTION

The recipe is mainly composed of drugs with warm and dry nature, so it is contraindicated in patients with convulsion due to endogenous wind.

218 JIUZHUAN HUANGJING DAN（九转黄精丹）

Pill of Siberian Solomonseal Rhizome

PRINCIPAL INGREDIENTS

Siberian solomonseal rhizome （Rhizoma Polygonati）, Chinese angelica root （Radix Angelicae Sinensis）

FUNCTIONS

Nourishing and strengthening the body.

INDICATIONS

Weakness of the body, sallow complexion and reducing of the appetite.

DIRECTIONS

To be taken orally, 1 pill each time , twice a day.

PRECAUTION

It is not advisable for cases of fever and sweat due to affection by exopathogen.

219 LIANGYI GAO（两仪膏）

Semifluid Extract of Pilose Asiabell Root and Fleece-flower Root

PRINCIPAL INGREDIENTS

Piloseasiabell root hen （Radix Codonopsis

Pilosulae), Fleece-flower root (Radix Polygoni Multiflori)

FUNCTIONS

Supplementing Qi and nourishing blood.

INDICATIONS

Deficiency of both Qi and blood, weakness
after illness.

DIRECTIONS

To be taken orally, 15g each time, twice a
day , take before meals.

PRECAUTION

Avoid raw, cold and greasy food.

220 GUISHAO LIUJUN WAN (归芍六君丸)

Pill of Angelica and Peony with Six Noble
Ingredients

PRINCIPAL INGREDIENTS

Chinese angelica root (Radix Angelicae),
White peony root (Radix Paeoniae Alba),
Pilose asiabell root (Radix Codonopsis Pilo-
sulae), Bighead atractylodes rhizome (Rhi-
zoma Atracty Ladis Macrocephalae), Poria
(Poria), Liquorice (Radix Glycyrrhizae),
Tangerine peel (Pericarpium Citri Reticu-
latae), Pinellia tuber (Rhizoma Pinelliae)

FUNCTIONS

Replenishing Qi and nourishing blood.

INDICATIONS

Unbalance between liver and spleen, abdominal distension and fullness, lassitude of extremities, vomiting.

DIRECTIONS

To be taken orally, 9g each time , twice a day.

PRECAUTION

Avold cold and greasy food.

221 QIBAO MEIRAN WAN (七宝美髯丸)

Tonic Bolus of Seven Precious Ingredients

PRINCIPAL INGREDIENTS

Fleece-flower root (Radix Polygoni Multiflori), Psoralea fruit (Fructus Psoraleae), Achyranthes and cyathula root (Radix Achyranthis Bidentoeet Radix Cyathulae), Chinese angelica root (Radix Angelicae Sinensis), Poria (Poria), Wolfberry fruit (Fructus Lycii), Dodder seed (Semen Cuscutae)

FUNCTIONS

Nourishing the liver and kidney, strengthening constitution and delaying senility.

INDICATIONS

Deficiency of both liver and kidney, early graying of hair, general debility of advanced age.

DIRECTIONS

To be taken orally, 1 bolus each time, twice a day.

PRECAUTION

Avoid cold and raw food.

222 YAN SHOU DAN (延寿丹)

Life-Prolonging Pill

PRINCIPAL INGREDIENTS

Fleece-flower root (Radix Polygoni Multiflori), Dried rehmannia root (Radix Rehmanniae), Honeysuckle flower (Flos Lonicerae), Eucommia bark (Cortex Eucommiae), Achyranthes and cyathula root (Radix Achyranthis Bidentae et Radix Cyathulae), Glossy privet fruit (Fructus Ligustri Lucici), Sesame seed (Semen Sesami), Eclipta (Herba Ecliptae), Dodder seed (Semen Cuscutae)

FUNCTIONS

Nourishing and tonifying liver and kidney, replenishing blood and vital essence.

INDICATIONS

Deficiency of the body, lassitude, dizziness. soreness in loins and weakeness of legs, importence, spermatorrhea.

DIRECTIONS

To be taken orally, 6g each time , twice a day.

PRECAUTION

It should be cautiously used for patients with cold and deficiency of spleen and stomach.

223 ZHUANGYAO JIANSHEN WAN（壮腰健肾丸）

Loins-Srengthening and Kidney-Invigorating Bolus

PRINCIPAL INGREDIENTS

Cibot rhizome (Rhizoma Cibotii), Cherokee rose-hip (Fructus Rosae Laevigatae), Scarlet kadsura root (Radix Kadsurae Coccineae), Loranthus mulberry mistletoe (Ramulus Loranthi), Spatholobus stem (Caulis Spatholobi), Dodder seed (Semen Cuscutae), Glossy privet fruit (Fructus Ligustri Lucidi), Siberian solomonseal rhizome (Rhizoma Polygonati), Prepared rehmannia root (Radix Rehmanniae Praeparata), Prepared fleece-flower root (Radix Polygoni Multiflori Praeparata)

FUNCTIONS

Strengthening loins, invigorating kidney,

dispelling pathogenic wind, removing dampness and activating the collaterals to relieve pain.

INDICATIONS

Lumbago due to deficiency of kidney,
arthralgia due to wind-dampness, weak
limbs, lassitude.

DIRECTIONS

To be taken orally, 1 bolus each time,
twice a day.

PRECAUTION

Not advisable for patients with fever due to
common cold.

224 DUHUO JISHENG WAN (独活寄生丸)

Pubescent Angelica and Loranthus Bolus

PRINCIPAL INGREDIENTS

Pubescent angelica root (Radix Angelicae
Pubescentis), Loranthus mulberry mistle-
toe (Ramulus Loranthi), Eucommia bark
(Cortex Eucommiae), Achyranthes root
(Radix Achyranthis Bidentatae), Wild gin-
ger (Herba Asari), Large-leaf gentian root
(Radix Gentianae Macrophyllae), Poria
(Poria), Cinnamon bark (Cortex Cinna-
moni), Ledebouriella root (Radix Lede-
bouriellae), Chuan xiong rhizome (Rhizoma

Ligustici Chuan xiong）, Ginseng（Radix Ginseng）, Licorice root （Radix Glycyrrhizae）, Chinese angelica root （Radix Angelicae Sinensis）, White peony root （Radix Paeoniae Alba）, Dried rehmannia root （Radix Rehmanniae）

FUNCTIONS

Dispelling wind-dampness, relieving pain due to arthralgia-syndrome, tonifying liver and kidney, invigorating Qi and nourishing the blood.

INDICATIONS

Persistent arthralgia-syndrome with deficiency of liver and kidney, marked by cold and pain of loins and knees, limited movement, soreness, weakness or numbness of the joints, etc.

DIRECTIONS

To be taken orally, 1 bolus each time, twice a day.

225　JIN GANG WAN（金刚丸）

Jingang Pill

PRINCIPAL INGREDIENTS

Desertliving cistanche （Herba Cistachis）, Eucommia bark （Cortex Eucommiae）, Dodder seed （Semen Cuscutae）, Seven-lobed yam (Rhizoma Dioscoreae Septemlobae)

FUNCTIONS

Tonifying liver and kidney , strengthening loins and knees.

INDICATIONS

Insufficiency of liver and kidney, malnutrition of bones and muscles, manifested as atrophic debilities, Bi syndromes, impotence, premature ejaculation.

DIRECTIONS

To be taken orally, 1 bolus each time , twice a day.

PRECAUTION

Avoid greasy food.

226 HU QIAN WAN (虎潜丸)

Strengthening Pill

PRINCIPAL INGREDIENTS

Tortoise plastron (Plastrum Testudinis), Prepared rehmannia root (Radix Rehmanniae Praeparata), Phellodendron bark (Cortex Phellodendri), Anemarrhena rhizome (Rhizoma Anemarrhenae), White peony root (Radix Paeoniae Alba), Cynomorium (Herba Cynomorii), Dried ginger (Rhizoma Zingiberis), Tangerine peel (Pericarpium Citri Reticalatae)

FUNCTIONS

Nourishing liver-Yin and kidney-Yin , strengthening muscles and bones.

INDICATIONS

Arthralgia-syndrome with deficiency of liver and kidney, marked by pain of bones and muscles. weakness and numbness of the joints.

DIRECTIONS

To be taken orally, 1 bolus each time, twice a day.

PRECAUTION

This recipe is contraindicated in atrophic debilities due to wind-cold-dampness.

227 WUZI YANZONG WAN (五子衍宗丸)

Multiplying Pill of Five Seeds

PRINCIPAL INGREDIENTS

Wolfberry fruit (Fructus Lycii), Dodder seed (Semen Cuscutae), Chinese raspberry (Fructus Rubi), Schisandra fruit (Fructus Schisandrae), Plantain seed (Semen Plantaginis)

FUNCTIONS

Tonifying kidney and invigorating the essence, strengthening kidney-Yang to treat emission.

INDICATIONS

Insufficiency of kidney-Qi, seminal emission, enuresis, soreness and weakness of loins and legs.

DIRECTIONS

To be taken orally, 1 bolus each time, 3 times a day.

PRECAUTION

It is forbidden to take greasy food.

228 WUBI SHANYAO WAN （无比山药丸）

Pill of Chinese Yam

PRINCIPAL INGREDIENTS

Dried rehmannia root (Radix Rehmanniae), Chinese yam (Rhizoma Dioscoreae), Red halloysite (Halloysitum Rubrum), Morinda root (Radix Morindae Officinalis), Poria (Poria), Achyranthes and cyathula root (Radix Achyranthis Bidentatae et Radix Cyathulae), Dogwood fruit (Fructus Corni), Oriental water plantain rhizome (Rhizoma Alismatis), Schisandra fruit (Fructus Schisandrae), Desertliving cistanche (Herba Cistachis), Dodder seed (Semen Cuscutae), Eucommia bark (Cortex Eucommiae)

FUNCTIONS

Strengthening spleen and nourishing kidney.

Deficiency of both spleen and kidney, poor appetite, general debility, weakness and soreness of loins and knees, vertigo tinnitus.

DIRECTIONS

To be taken orally, 9g each time, twice a day.

229   GUILU ERJIAO WAN（龟鹿二胶丸）

Tonic Bolus with Tortoise Plastron and Anter Glue

PRINCIPAL INGREDIENTS

Tortoise-plastron glue (Colla Plastri Testudinis), Antler glue (Colla Cornus Cervi), Prepared rehmannia root (Radix Rehmanniae Praeparata), Chinese yam (Rhizoma Dioscoreae), Poria (Poria), Eucommia bark (Cortex Eucommiae), Oriental water Plantain rhizome (Rhizoma Alismatis), Moutan bark (Cortex Moutan Radicis), Cinnamon bark (Cortex Cinnamomi), Chinese angelica root (Radix Angelicae Sinensis), White peony root (Radix Paeoniae Alba), Wolfberry fruit (Fructus Lycii), Schisandra fruit (Fructus Schisandrae),

Psoralea fruit (Fructus Psoraleae)

FUNCTIONS

Warming and tonifying the kidney-Yang, nourishing the vital essence.

INDICATIONS

Insufficiency of the kidney-Yang, deficiency of vital essence and blood manifested by impotence, lassitude in the lions, diabetes, dizziness, etc.

DIRECTIONS

To be taken orally, 6g each time, twice a day.

PRECAUTION

It is forbidden to take cool food.

230 HECHE DAZAO WAN (河车大造丸)

Restorative Bolus with Human Placenta

PRINCIPAL INGREDIENTS

Human Placenta, Prepared rehmannia root (Radix Rehmanniae Praeparata), Lucid asparagi (Radix Asparagi), Ophiopogon root (Radix Opiopogonics), Tortoise plastron (Plastrum Testudinis), Phellodendron bark (Cortex Phellodendri), Eucommia bark (Cortex Eucommitae), Achyranthes and cyathula root (Radix Achyranthis Bidentae et Radix Cyathulae)

FUNCTIONS

Nourishing Yin and enriching blood, tonifying Lung and strengthening kidney.

INDICATIONS

Insufficiency of blood and vital essence, deficiency of Lung-Yin and kidney-Yin, marked as general debility, hectic fever, night sweat, cough, soreness and weakness of loins and knees.

DIRECTIONS

To be taken orally, 1 bolus each time, twice a day.

PRECAUTION

It is not advisable for patients of deficiency of spleen and stomach, poor appetite, watery stool, etc.

231 SHEN QI CHONGJI (参芪冲剂)

Infusion of Ginseng and Astragalus

PRINCIPAL INGREDIENTS

Ginseng (Radix Ginseng), Aconthopanax root (Radix Acanthopanacis Senticosi), Astragalus root (Radix Astragaliseu Hedysari), Red peony root (Radix Paeoniae Rubra), Cinnamon twig (Ramulus Cinnamomi)

FUNCTIONS

Promoting blood circulation to remove blood stasis , replenishing Qi and restoring pulse.

INDICATIONS

Headache, dizziness, numbness of limbs, difficulty in walking and others caused by blood stasis due to Qi deficiency .

DIRECTIONS

To be taken orally after being infused in boiling water, 12~24g each time , twice a day.

232 ZIHECHE FEN (紫河车粉)

Powder of Human Placenta

PRINCIPAL INGREDIENTS

Human placenta

FUNCTIONS

Invigorating Qi and nourishing blood.

INDICATIONS

Insuffiiency of both Qi and blood, marked as magersucht and lassitude of the body, mental fatigue, pale complexion, palpitation, spontaneous perspiration, night sweat, weakness after delivery.

DIRECTIONS

To be taken orally, 3g each time , 1 or 2 times a day.

PRECAUTION

It is contraindicated to patients of affection by exopathogen.

233 GENG NIAN AN （更年安）

Climacteric Syndrome Relieving Tablet

PRINCIPAL INGREDIENTS

Prepared rehmannia root (Radix Rehmanniae Praeparata）, Fleece-flower root (Radix Polygoni Multiflori）, Oriental water plantain (Rhizoma Alismatis）, Poria (Poria）, Schisandra fruit (Fructus Schisandrae）, Pearl shell (Concha Margaritifera Usta）, Fleece-flower stem (Caulis Polygoni Multiflori）, Scrophularia root (Radix Scrophulariae）, Light wheat (Fructus Tritici Levis)

FUNCTIONS

Nourishing Yin and clearing away heat, relieving restlessness and tranquilizing mind.

INDICATIONS

Female climacteric syndrome, marked by tidal fever with sweating, vertigo, insomnia, dysphoriairrilability, fluctuation of blood pressure.

DIRECTIONS

To be taken orally, 6 tablets each time, 2～ 3 times a day.

It is not advisable for patients with cold extremities, and aversion to cold due to insufficiency of spleen-Yang and kidney-Yang.

234 GUILU ERXIAN GAO (龟鹿二仙膏)

Semifluid Extract of Tortoise Plastron and Antler Glue

PRINCIPAL INGREDIENTS

Tortoise plastron (Plastrum Testudinis), Antler glue (Colla Cornus Cervi), Ginseng (Radix Ginseng), Wolfberry fruit (Fructus Lycii)

FUNCTIONS

Supplementing Qi and nourishing blood, nourishing Yin and strengthening Yang.

INDICATIONS

Deficiency of Kidney-Qi, soreness and pain in loins and back, seminal emission, vertigo.

DIRECTIONS

To be taken orally, 10g each time , 3 times a day.

PRECAUTION

Contraindicated to exopathic disease.

235 ZHENQI FUZHENG CHONGJI (贞芪扶

正冲剂）

Infusion of Astragalus Root and Glossy Privet

PRINCIPAL INGREDIENTS

Astragalus root （Radix Astragali Seu Hedysari）, Glossy privet (Fructus Ligustri Lucici)

FUNCTIONS

Tonifying and strengthening both Yin and Yang, reinforcing body resistance.

INDICATIONS

Deficiency of both Qi and Yin, manifested as dizziness, tinnitus, short breath, chest distress, sweating, mental fatigue, pale tongue with white fur, deep, thready and weak pulse.

DIRECTIONS

To be taken orally after being infused in boiling water, 15g each time , 3 times a day.

PRECAUTION

Contraindicated to raw cold and greasy food.

I -13 Prescriptions for Inducing Resuscitation
开窍剂

236 ANGONG NIUHUANG WAN （安宫牛黄丸）

Bezoar Bolus for Resurrection

PRINCIPAL INGREDIENTS

Cow-bezoare （Calulus Bovis）, Musk （Moschus）, Goldthread root （Rhizoma Coptidis）, Scutellaria root （Radix Scutellariae）, Borneol （Borneolum）, Curcuma root （Radix Curcumae）, Pearl （Margarita）, Realgar （Realgar）, Gold foil （Appropriate amount）

FUNCTIONS

Clearing away heat and toxins and eliminating phlegm to induce resuscitation.

INDICATIONS

Attack of pericardium by pathogenic heat occurring in the course of epidemic febrile diseases or accumulation of phlegm-heat in the heart manifested as high fever, dysphasia, coma and delirium or coma due to apoplexy, infantile convulsion and so on.

DIRECTIONS

To be taken orally, 3g each time, 2 ~ 3 times a day.

PRECAUTION

It should be cautiously used in deficiency case.

237 JUFANG ZHIBAO DAN（局方至宝丹）

Jufang Treasured Bolus

PRINCIPAL INGREDIENTS

Musk （Moschus）, Borneol （Borneolum）,
Benzoin （Benzoinum）, Cow-bezoare （Cal-
culus Bovis）, Tortoise shell （Carapax Eret-
mochelydis）, Amber （Succinum）, Realgar
（Realgar）

FUNCTIONS

Eliminating turbid pathogenic factor to induce resuscitation and clearing away heat
and toxins.

INDICATIONS

Stagnation of Phlegm-heat in the interior
marked by coma and delirium, feverish
body and irritability, abundant expectoration, harsh respiration, red tongue with
yellow, thick and greasy fur, slippery and
rapid pulse, and infantile convulsion associated with the above syndrome.

DIRECTIONS

To be taken orally, 1.5g each time, 2～3
times a day.

PRECAUTION

It should not be used for a long time.

WANSHI NIUHUANG QINGXINWAN
（万氏牛黄清心丸）

Bolus of Cow-Bezoar for Clearing Heart-Fire

PRINCIPAL INGREDIENTS

Artificia cow-bezoar (Calculus Bovis Artificiosus), Curcuma (Radix Curcumae), Capejasmine (Fructus Gardenias), Coptis root (Rhizoma Coptidis), Scutellaria root (Radix Scutellariae)

FUNCTIONS

Removing heat from the heart to restore consciousness and reducing heat and eliminating phlegm for resuscitation.

INDICATIONS

The accumulation of heat-phlegm in the body, and the attack of pericardium by heat, manifested as stroke, coma, delirium, restlessness, wheezing sound and abundant expectoration, high fever and convulsion.

DIRECTIONS

To be taken orally, with warm boiled water, 1~2 boluses each time, twice a day.

PRECAUTION

Never administered to patients with deficiency syndrome.

239 QINGKAILING ZHUSHEYE （清开灵注射液）

Injection for Clearing away Heat

PRINCIPAL INGREDIENTS

Buffalo horn （Cornu Bubali）, Scutellaria root （Radix Scutellariae）, Isatis root （Radix Isatidis）, Capejasmine fruit （Fructus Gardeniae）, Honeysuckle flower （Flos Lonicerae）

FUNCTIONS

Clearing away heat to restore consciousness.

INDICATIONS

Attack of pericardium by pathogenic heat, manifested as high fever, dysphorsia, coma and delirium, irritability, convulsion, etc..

DIRECTIONS

To be used by injection, 2～4ml each time, 2～3 times a day.

PRECAUTION

Contraindicated to patients of high fever together with shock, or low blood pressure.

240 SUHEXIANG WAN （苏合香丸）

Storax Pill

PRINCIPAL INGREDIENTS

Oriental sweetgum resin (Resina Liquidambaris Orientalix), Mask (Moschus), Borneol (Borneolum), Benzoin (Benzoinum), Dutchmanspipe root (Radix Aristolochiae), White scandal wood (Lignum Santali), Eagle wood (Lignum Aquilariae Resinatum), Cloves (Flos Caryophylli), Nutgrass flatsedge rhizome (Rhizoma Cyperi), Obibanum (Resina Olibani), Long pepper (Fructus Piperis Longi), Bighead atractylodes rhizome (Rhizoma Atractylodis Macrocephalae), Myrobalan fruit (Fructus Chebulae)

FUNCTIONS

Inducing resuscitation with aromatics, promoting the circulation of Qi to relieve pain.

INDICATIONS

Cold syndrome of coma marked by sudden fainting, trismus, unconsciousness, or fullness with cold sensation in the chest and abdomen, nausea and so on.

DIRECTIONS

To be taken orally, 1 bolus each time , 1～2 times a day.

PRECAUTION

It is advisable for pregnant women.

241　GUANXIN SUHE WAN（冠心苏合丸）

Storax Pill for Treating Coronary Heart Disease

PRINCIPAL INGREDIENTS

Storax（Styrax），Borneol（Borneolum），Frankincense（Resina Oblibani），Sandalwood（Lignum Santali），Dutchmanspipe root（Radix Aristolochiae）

FUNCTIONS

Regulating the flow of Qi and soothing chest oppression，promoting blood circulation to relieve pain.

INDICATIONS

Angina pectoris，chest distress and short breath.

DIRECTIONS

To be masticated，1 pill each time ，3 times a day.

PRECAUTION

Never administered to pregnant women.

242　SHIXIANG FANSHENG DAN（十香返生丹）

Lifesaving Pill with Ten Kinds of Fragrant Drugs

PRINCIPAL INGREDIENTS

Oriental sweetgum（Resina Liquidambayis

Orientalis). Musk (Moschus). Benzoin
(Benzoinum). Borneol (Borneolum). Dutc-
hmanspipe root (Radix Aristolochiae).
White sandal wood (Lignum Santali). Ea-
gle wood (Lignum Aquilariae Resinatum).
Cloves (Flos Caryophylli). Nutgrass
flatsedge rhizome (Rhizoma Cyperi).
Olibanum (Resina dibani). Myrobalan fruit
(Fructus Chebulae). Gastrodia tuber (Rhi-
zoma Gastrodiae). Liquorice (Radix Gly-
cyrrhizae). Curcuma root (Radix
Curcumae). Trichosanthes fruit (Fructus
Trichosanthis). Lotus seed (Semen
Nelumbinis)

FUNCTIONS

Inducing resuscitation with aromatics, resolving phlegm and relieving convulsion.

INDICATIONS

Coma and syncope, infantile convulsion
trismus, unconsciousness, etc.

DIRECTIONS

To be taken orally, 1 bolus each time,
twice a day.

PRECAUTION

Pregnant women are forbidden to use the
recipe.

243 XINGNAO JIANGYA WAN (醒脑降压丸)

Consciousness-Restoring and Antihypertensive Pill

PRINCIPAL INGREDIENTS

Coptis root (Rhizoma Coptidis), Scutellaria root (Radix Scutellariae), Curcuma root (Radix Curcumae), Capejasmine fruit (Fructus Gardeniae), Borneol (Borneolum), Magnolia flower (Flos Magnoliae)

FUNCTIONS

Clearing away heat and purging fire, tranquilizing the mind, inducing resuscitation.

INDICATIONS

Dizziness, headache, insomnia, palpitation, etc..

DIRECTIONS

To be taken orally, 5 ~ 10 boluses each time, 1~2 times a day.

PRECAUTION

Contraindicated for pregnant women.

I -14 Prescriptions for Tranquilization
安神剂

244 BAIZI YANGXIN WAN (柏子养心丸)

Mind-Easing Tonic Bolus with Arborvitae Seed

PRINCIPAL INGREDIENTS

Arborvitae seed (Semen Biotae), Pilose asiabell root (Radix Codonopsis Pilosulae), Astragalus root (Radix Astragali seu Hedysari), Chuanxiong rhizome (Rhizoma Ligustici Chuanxiong), Chinese angelica root (Radix Angelicae Sinensis), Poria (Poria), Polygala root (Radix Polygalae), Spiny date seed (Semen Ziziphi Spinisae), Cinnamon bark (Cortex Cinnamomi), Schisandra fruit (Fructus Schisandrae), Pinellia tuber leaven (Rhizoma Pinelliae Fermentatum), Liquorice (Radix Glycyrrhizae)

FUNCTIONS

Replenishing Qi, nourishing blood and tranquilizing mind.

INDICATIONS

Insufficiency of heart-Qi, manifested as short breath, aversion to cold, emotional distress, insomnia, amnesia, nightmare, severe palpitation due to fright, etc.

DIRECTIONS

To be taken orally, 1 bolus each time, twice a day.

245 ZHENZHONG WAN (枕中丸)

Zhenzhong Pill

PRINCIPAL INGREDIENTS

Tortoise plastron (Plastrum Testudinis),
Dragon's bone (Os Craconis Fossilia),
Grassleaved sweetflag rhizome (Rhizoma A-
cori Graminei), Polygala root (Radix Polygalae)

FUNCTIONS

Nourishing Yin and clearing fire, regulating
heart and kidney.

INDICATIONS

Dysphoria, insomnia, palpitation, frequent
dreams, spermatorrhea, etc.

DIRECTIONS

To be taken orally, 1 bolus each time , 2~
3 times a day.

PRECAUTION

Contraindicated for patients of deficiency of
both spleen and stomach, poor appetite,
watery stool.

246 JIAOTAI WAN (交泰丸)

Pill for Regulating Heart and Kidney

PRINCIPAL INGREDIENTS

Coptis root (Rhizoma Coptidis), Cinnamon
bark (Cortex Cinnamomi)

FUNCTIONS

Regulating heart and kidney.

INDICATIONS

Disharmony between heart and kidney, marked by dysphoria, insomnia, palpitation, frequent dreams, spermatorrhea, etc.

DIRECTIONS

To be taken orally, 2～3g each time, 2～3 times a day.

PRECAUTION

Contraindicated for patients of insomnia due to Yin-deficiency.

247　ZHENHE LING PIAN (珍合灵片)

Tranquilizing Tablet with Pearl

PRINCIPAL INGREDIENTS

Pearl (Margarita), Lucid ganoderma (Ganoderma Lucidum), Licorice root (Radix Glycyrrhizae)

FUNCTIONS

Relieving palpitation and tranquilizing the mind, nourishing and reinforcing five parenchymatous viscera.

INDICATIONS

Palpitation, insomnia.

DIRECTIONS

To be taken orally, 3～4 tablets each time, 3 times a day.

Patients with deficiency of heart-Yang and kidney-Yang should be prudent when using the recipe.

248　FUBO ANSHEN WAN（琥珀安神丸）

Amber Sedative Pill

PRINCIPAL INGREDIENTS

Amber (Succinum), Dried rehmannia root (Radix Rehmanniae), Figwort root (Radix Scrophulariae), Red sage root (Radix Salviae Miltiorrhizae), Chinese angelica root (Radix Angelicae Sinensis), Ginseng (Radix Ginseng), Poria (Poria), Arborvitae seed (Semen Biotae), Wild or sping jujuba seed (Semen Ziziphi Spinosae), Plolygala asparagus root (Radix Polygalae), Lucid root (Radix Asparagi), Lilyturf root (Radix Ophiopogonis), Magnolia vine fruit (Fructus Schisandrae), Root of balloon-flower (Radix Platycodi), Dragon's bone (Os Craconis Fossilia), Liquorice (Radix Glycyrrhizae), Albizia bark (Flos Albiziae), Chinese date (Fructus Ziziphi Jujubae)

FUNCTIONS

Nourishing Yin to remove heat, tranquilizing the mind.

INDICATIONS

Insufficiency of both heart and kidney，
manifested as insomnia，palpitation，mental
irritability，amnesia，spermatorrhea，etc.

DIRECTIONS

To be taken orally，1 bolus each time ，
twice a day.

PRECAUTION

The recipe is composed of greasy drugs，
which affect stomach，so it is not fit to take
for a long time.

I -15 Prescriptions for Inducing Astringency
固涩剂

249 JINSUO GUJING WAN （金锁固精丸）

Golden Lock Pill for Keeping the Kidney
Essence

PRINCIPAL INGREDIENTS

Flatstem milkvetch seed （Semen Astragali
complanti），Gordon euryale （Semen Eur-
yales），Lotus stamen （Stamen Nelum-
binis），Lotus seed （Semen Nelumbinis），
Dragon's bone （Os Draconis Fossilia Ossis
Mastodi），Oyster shell （Concha Ostreae）

FUNCTIONS

Consolidating kidney to treat emission.

INDICATIONS

Unconsolidation of the essence gate due to deficiency of the kidney manifested as emission, spermatorrhea, lumbago, tinnitus, lassitude, pale tongue with white fur, thready and feeble pulse.

DIRECTIONS

To be taken orally, 3 ~ 6g each time, 3 times a day.

PRECAUTION

Contraindicated for patients with emission due to downward flow of damp-heat from liver channel or hyperactivity of pathogenic fire due to Yin deficiency.

250 JINYINGZI GAO（金樱子膏）

Semifluid Extracts of Cherokee Rose-Hip

PRINCIPAL INGREDIENT

Cherokee rose-hip （Fructus Rosae Laevigatae）

FUNCTIONS

Astringing the kidney to arrest spontaneous emission.

INDICATIONS

Insufficiency of both spleen and kidney, instability of the kidney manifested as emission, lumbago, tinnitus, spermatorrhea, lassitude, etc.

DIRECTIONS

To be taken orally, 15g each time, 3 times a day.

PRECAUTION

Avoid greasy food.

251 SUOQUAN WAN (缩泉丸)

Pill for Reducing Urination

PRINCIPAL INGREDIENTS

Bitter cardamon (Fructus Alpiniae Oxyphyllae), Lindera root (Radix Linderae), Chinese yam (Rhizoma Dioscoreae)

FUNCTIONS

Warming and reinforcing spleen and kidney, keeping the kidney essence and reducing urination.

INDICATIONS

Insufficiency of spleen-Yang and kidney-Yang, manifested as seminal emission, enuresis, dribbling urination, frequent nocturnal urination, etc.

DIRECTIONS

To be taken orally, 9g each time, twice a day.

PRECAUTION

It should be cautiously for patients with damp heat.

252 ANGONG JIANGYA WAN（安宫降压丸）

Resurrecting and Antihypertensive Pill

PRINCIPAL INGREDIENTS

Cow bezoar (Calculus Bovis)，Buffalo horn (Cornu Bubali)，Gastrodia tuber（Rhizoma Gastrodiae)，Curcuma root (Radix Curcumae)，Borneol (Borneolum)

FUNCTIONS

Clearing heart and cooling liver，checking endogenous wind，calming the liver and suppressing hyperactivity of liver-Yang.

INDICATIONS

Hyperactivity of liver-Yang，headache，dizziness，dysphoria，palpitation，irritability，etc.

DIRECTIONS

To be taken orally，1～2 bolus each time，twice a day.

PRECAUTION

Avoid over-dosage.

253 NAO LI QING（脑立清）

Tranquilizing Bolus

PRINCIPAL INGREDIENTS

Red ochre (Ochra Haematitum), Magnetite (Magnetium), Pearl (Margarita), Borneol (Borneolum), Achyranthes and cyathula root (Radix Achyranthis Bidentatae et Radix Cyathulae), Pinellia tuber (Rhizoma Pinelliae), Peppermint (Herba Menthae), Medicated leaven (Massa Fermentata Medicinalis)

FUNCTIONS

Clearing heat and calming the liver, suppressing sthenic Yang and tranquilizing the mind.

INDICATIONS

Hyperactivity of liver-Yang, dizziness, tinnitus, dry throat and mouth, insomnia with vexation, red tongue with yellow fur, taut pulse.

DIRECTIONS

To be taken orally, 10 boluses each time, twice a day.

254　ZIXUE SAN（紫雪散）

Purple Snowy Powder

PRINCIPAL INGREDIENTS

Musk (Muschus), Antelope's horn (Cornu Saigae Tataricae), Cypsum (Cypsum Fibro-

sum), Calcite (Cakitum), Tale (Talcum),
Magnetite (Magnetitum), Costus root (Radix Aucklandiae), Gloves (Flos Caryophylli), Eaglewood (Lignum Aquilariae Resinatum)

FUNCTIONS

Clearing away heat and toxic materials, and eliminating pathogenic wind to arrest convulsion.

INDICATIONS

Symptoms caused by febrile diseases such as high fever, restlessness, convulsion, maculopapule caused by noxious heat, coma and delirium, mania, stiff neck.

DIRECTIONS

To be taken orally, 1.5g each time, twice a day.

PRECAUTION

Contraindicated for patients in pregnancy.

255 NIUHUANG QINGXIN WAN (牛黄清心丸)

Cow-Bezoar Sedative Bolus

PRINCIPAL INGREDIENTS

Chinese yam (Rhizoma Dioscoreae), Ginseng (Radix Ginseng), Bighead atractylodes rhizome (Rhizoma Atroctylodis Mac-

rocephalae), Chinese angelica root (Radix
Angelicae Sinensis), White peony root
(Radix Paeoniae Alba), Antelope's horn
(Cornu Saigae Tataticae), Artificialcow-be-
zoar (Calculus Bovis Facticius), Musk
(Muschus)

FUNCTIONS

Supplementing Qi, nourishing blood, tranquilizing the mind, allaying excitement and
eliminating phlegm for resuscitation.

INDICATIONS

Stagnated heat in the chest, palpitation due
to fright, fidgeting due to deficiency, vertigo, aphasia from apoplexy, deviation of the
eye and mouth, hemiplegia, dysphasia and
vague mind caused by deficiency of Qi and
blood as well as upward disturbance of
phlegm and heat.

DIRECTIONS

To be taken orally, 1 bolus each time, 2 boluses for serious case, twice a day.

PRECAUTION

Contraindicated for pregnant women.

256 HUITIAN ZAIZAO WAN（回天再造丸）

Restorative Bolus with Tremendous Powder

PRINCIPAL INGREDIENTS

Ginseng (Rdaix Ginseng), Cow-bozear (Calculus Bovis), Musk (Moschus), Gastrodia tuber (Rhizoma Gastrodiae), Dragon's blood (Resina Draconis), Rhinoceros horn (Cornu Rhinocerotis), Goral blood (Sanguis Naemorhedi)

FUNCTIONS

Dispelling wind, resolving phlegm and promoting blood circulation to remove obstruction in the channels.

INDICATIONS

Hemiplegia, facial hemiparalysis, soreness in loins and legs, numbness of limbs.

DIRECTIONS

To be taken orally, 1 bolus each time, twice a day.

PRECAUTION

Contraindicated for pregnant women.

257 TIANMA SHOUWU WAN (天麻首乌丸)

Tablet of Gastrodia Tuber and Fleece-Flower Root

PRINCIPAL INGREDIENTS

Gastrodia tuber (Rhizoma Gastrodiae), Tribulus fruit (Fructus Tribuli), Fleece-flower root (Radix Polygoni Multiflori),

Chuanxiong rhizome (Rhizoma Chuanxiong), Eclipta (Herba Ecliptae)

FUNCTIONS

Nourishing and reinforcing liver and kidney, checking endogenous wind and improving acuity of vision.

INDICATIONS

Insufficiency of liver-Yin and kidney-Yin,
hyperactivity of liver-Yang, marked as
dizziness, headache, tinnitus, soreness and
weakness in loins and knees etc.

DIRECTIONS

To be taken orally, 6 tablets each time, 3
times a day.

PRECAUTION

Avoid pungent and greasy food during the
administration.

I -17 Prescriptions for Expelling Worms
驱虫剂

258 WUMEI WAN (乌梅丸)

Black Plum Pill

PRINCIPAL INGREDIENTS

Black plum (Fructus Mume), Coptis root
(Rhizoma Coptidis), Phellodendron bark
(Cortex Phellodendri), Dried ginger (Rhi-

zoma Zingiberis), Cinnamon twig (Ramulus Cinnamomi), Prepared lateral root of a-conite (Radix Aconiti Lateralis Prae-parata), Chinese angelica root (Radix An-gelicae Sinensis), Ginseng (Radix Ginseng), Asarum herb (Herba Asari)

FUNCTIONS

Relieving colic caused by ascaris.

INDICATIONS

Colic caused by ascaris.

DIRECTIONS

To be taken orally, 1 bolus each time, 3 times a day.

PRECAUTION

Contraindicated for pregnant women.

259 FUFANG ZHEGU SAN (复方鹧鸪散)

Compound Powder of Chinese Francolin

PRINCIPAL INGREDIENTS

Chinese francclin (Partridge), Levomycetin

FUNCTIONS

Expelling ascaris.

INDICATIONS

Ascariasis.

DIRECTIONS

To be taken orally, for 1 year old, 1 pocket each time; 2~3 years old, 1.5 pockets each

time; 4~6 years old, 2 pockets each time;
7~8 years old, 3 pockets each time; 10~14
years old, 4 pockets each time; over 14
years old, 5 pockets each time, once a day.

PRECAUTION

It should not be over used for children

260 WENJING WAN （温经丸）

Pill for Warming Channels

PRINCIPAL INGREDIENTS

Evodia Fruit (Fructus Evodiae), Cinnamon twig （Ramulus Cinnamomi）, Chinese angelica root （Radix Angelicae Sinensis）, Chuan-xiong rhizome （Rhizoma Ligustici Chuanxiong）, Peony root （Radix Paeoniae）, Licorice root （Radix Glycyrrhizae）, Donkey-hide gelatin （Colla Corii Asini）, Lilyturf root （Radix Ophiopogonis）, Moutan bark （Cortex Moutan Radicis）, Ginseng （Radix Ginseng）, Pinellia tuber （Rhizoma Pinelliae）, Fresh ginger （Rhizoma Zingiberis Recens）

FUNCTIONS

Warming the channels and expelling cold, nourishing the blood and dispelling blood stasis.

INDICATIONS

Irregular menstruation due to the deficiency-cold in the Chong and Ren channels and accumulation of stagnant blood, marked by preceded or delayed menstrual cycle, or overdue or persistent menstrual duration, or occurrence of menstruation twice or more in one month, or nightfall fever, feverish sensation in the palms, parched lips and dry mouth, pain and cold in the lower abdomen, failure to conceive for a long time.

DIRECTIONS

To be taken orally, 1 bolus each time, twice a day.

PRECAUTION

It is forbidden for patients who have the syndrome of blood heat with blood stasis.

261 AIFU NUANGONG WAN （艾附暖宫丸）

Uterus-Warming Pill with Argyi Leaf and Evodia Fruit

PRINCIPAL INGREDIENTS

Argyi leaf （Folium Artemisiae Argyi）, Evodia fruit （Fructus Evodiae）, Cinnamon bark （Cortex Cinnamomi）, Astragalus root （Radix Astragali seu Hedysari）, Chinese angelica root （Radix Angelicae Sinensis）, White Peony root （Radix Paeoniae Alba）, Chuanxiong rhizome （Rhizoma Ligustici Chuanxiong）, Dried rehmannia root （Radix

Rehmanniae), Cyperus tuber (Rhizoma
Cyperi), Dipsacus root (Radix Dipsaci)

FUNCTIONS

Warming the uterus, regulating menstruation.

INDICATIONS

Accumulation of stagnant blood due to deficiency-cold in the uterus, marked by dys-
nenorrhea, irregular menstruation, delayed
menstrual cycle, failure to conceive for a
long time.

DIRECTIONS

To be taken orally, 1 bolus each time,
twice a day.

PRECAUTION

Contraindicated for patients with sthenic
heat differentiation.

262　SIZHI XIANGFU WAN（四制香附丸）

Cyperus Tuber Pill

PRINCIPAL INGREDIENTS

Cyperus tuber (Rhizoma Cyperi), Chuanxiong rhizome (Rhizoma Ligustici Chuanxiong), White peony root (Radix Paeoniae
Alba), Liquorice (Radix Glycyrrhizae),
Tangerine peel (Pericarpium Citri Reticulatae), White atractylodes rhizome (Rhi-

zoma Atractylodis Macrocephalae), Prepared rehmannia root (Radix Rehmanniae Praeparata), Phellodendron bark (Cortex Phellodendri)

FUNCTIONS

Nourishing the blood to regulate menstruation, regulating Qi and activating blood circulation.

INDICATIONS

Irregular menstruation, dysmenorrhea, pain and distension in the hypochondrium, taut pulse.

DIRECTIONS

To be taken orally, 1 bolus each time, 3 times a day.

PRECAUTION

Avoid cool food.

263 YIMUCAO LIUJIN GAO (益母草流浸膏)

Semifluid Extract of Motherwort

PRINCIPAL INGREDIENT

Motherwort (Herba Leonuri)

FUNCTIONS

Promoting blood circulation and removing blood stasis, nourishing the blood and regulating menstruation.

INDICATIONS

Irregular or stagnant menstruation, distending pain in the lower abdomen, amenorrhea, postpartum abdominal pain due to blood stasis.

DIRECTIONS

To be taken orally, 5~10ml each time, 2~3 times a day.

PRECAUTION

Contraindicated for patients in pregnancy.

264 FUKANGNING PIAN (妇康宁片)

Tablet for Women's Health and Tranquilness

PRINCIPAL INGREDIENTS

Chinese angelica root (Radix Angelicae Sinensis), Notoginseng (Radix Notoginseng), White peony root (Radix Paeoniae Alba), Motherwort (Herba Leonuri), Nutgrass flatsedge rhizome (Rhizoma Cyperi)

FUNCTIONS

Regulating menstruation, replenishing blood and regulating Qi to relieve pain.

INDICATIONS

Stagnancy of Qi and blood stasis manifested as dysmenorrhea, amenorrhea, metrorrhagia and metrostaxis, abdominal pain after delivery, persistent lochia and so on.

DIRECTIONS

To be taken orally, 8 tablets each time, 2~3 times a day.

PRECAUTION

Contraindicated for patients in pregnancy.

265 DINGKUN DAN (定坤丹)

Bolus for Woman Diseases

PRINCIPAL INGREDIENTS

Chinese angelica root (Radix Angelicae Sinensis), Ginseng (Radix Ginseng), Prepared rehmannia root (Radix Rehmanniae Praeparata), Pilose antler (Cornu cervi Pantotrichum), Bighead atractylodes rhizome (Rhizoma Atractylodis Macrocephalae), Poria (Poria), Eucommia bark (Cortex Eucommiae), Nutgrass flatsedge rhizome (Rhizoma Cyperi), Amomum fruit (Fructus Amomi), Corydalis tuber (Rhizoma Corydalis)

FUNCTIONS

Replenishing Qi and nourishing the blood, regulating menstruation by eliminating stagnation of Qi, warming the uterus and stopping metrorrhagia.

INDICATIONS

Menoxenia, menorrhalgia, deficiency of

both Qi and the blood, metrorrhagia or
metrostaxis, leukorrhagia, cold sensation in
the abdomen, tight feeling in the waist,
hectic fever, tuberculosis marked by deficiency of blood, postparturm deficiency.

DIRECTIONS

To be taken orally, half or one pill each
time, twice a day.

PRECAUTION

Avoid raw, cold, greasy and other irritating
foods. It is not advisable for those who
have got a cold.

266 TONGJING WAN (痛经丸)

Pill for Eliminating Dysmenorrhea

PRINCIPAL INGREDIENTS

Chinese agelica root (Radix Angelicae Sinen-
sis), Baked ginger (Rhizoma Zingiberis),
Cinnamon bark (Cortex Cinnamomi),
Cyperus tuber (Rhizoma Cyperi), Aucklan-
dia root (Radix Aucklandiae), Red sage root
(Radix Salviae Miltiorrhizae), Safflower
(Flos Carthami), Hawthorn fruit (Fructus
Crataegi), Motherwort (Herba Leonuri),
Corydalis tuber (Rhizoma Corydalis),
White peony root (Radix Paeoniae
Sinensis), Chuanxiong rhizome (Rhizoma

Ligustici Chuanxiong)

FUNCTIONS

Promoting the flow of Qi and blood circulation, expelling coldness to relieve pain.

INDICATIONS

Irregular menstruation, dysmenorrhea due to stagnation of Qi, accumulation of pathogenic cold, and obstruction of blood.

DIRECTIONS

To be taken orally, 6~9g each time, twice a day.

PRECAUTION

Contraindicated for patients with pregnancy.

267 BAZHEN YIMU WAN（八珍益母丸）

Eight Precious Ingredients Pill with Matherwort

PRINCIPAL INGREDIENTS

Pilose asiabell root (Radix Codonopsis Pilosulae), Bighead atractylodes rhizome (Rhizoma Atractylodis Macrocephalae), Poria (Poria), Liquorice (Radix Glycyrrhizae), Chinese angelica root (Radix Angelicae Sinensis), Chuanxiong rhizome (Rhizoma Ligustici Chuanxiong), White peony root (Radix Paeoniae Alba), Prepared rehman-

nia root (Radix Rehmanniae Praeparata),
Motherwort (Herba Leonuri)

FUNCTIONS

Invigorating Qi and blood, nourishing blood
to regulate menstruation.

INDICATIONS

Deficiency of both Qi and blood, manifested
as delay menstruation, amenorrhea, or
scanty menstruation, sallow complexion,
poor appetite, mental fatigue and tiredness,
short breath, palpitation, dizziness.

DIRECTIONS

To be taken orally, 1 bolus each time, 3
times a day.

PRECAUTION

Avoid raw, cold foods and cool or cold
drugs.

268   WUJI BAIFENG WAN (乌鸡白凤丸)

White Phoenix Bolus of Black-Bone Chick-
en

PRINCIPAL INGREDIENTS

Black-bone chicken (Gallus Domesticus),
Antler glue (Colla Cornus Cervi), Turtle
shell (Carapax Trionycis), Oyster shell
(Concha Ostreae), Mantis egg-case (Oo-
theca Mantidis), Ginseng (Radix Gin-

seng), Astragalus root (Radix Astragali seu Hedysari), Chinese angelica root (Radix Angelicae Sinensis), White peony root (Radix Paeoniae Alba), Nutgrass flatsedge rhizome (Rhizoma Cyperi), Lucid asparagus root (Radix Asparagi), Liquorice (Radix Glycyrrhizae), Rehmannia root (Radix Rehmanniae), Prepared rehmannia root (Radix Rehmanniae Praeparata), Chuanxiong rhizome (Rhizoma Ligustici Chuanxiong), Stellaria root (Radix Stellariae), Red sage root (Radix Salviae Miltiorrhizae), Chinese yam (Rhizoma Dioscoreae), Gordon euryale seed (Semen Euryales), Deglued anttler powder (Cornu Cervi Degelatinatum)

FUNCTIONS

Replenshing Qi and nourishing blood, regulating menstruation and arresting leukorrhagia.

INDICATIONS

Deficiency of both Qi and blood, pathological leanness and weakness, aching and weak loins and knees, irregular menstruation, metrorrhagia and metrostaxis, leukorrhagia.

DIRECTIONS

To be taken orally, 1 bolus each time, twice a day.

PRECAUTION

Avoid raw and cold food.

269 BABAO KUNSHUN WAN（八宝坤顺丸）

Pill for Regulating Menstruation

PRINCIPAL INGREDIENTS

Motherwort (Herba Leonuri), Chinese angelica root (Radix Angelicae Sinensis), Dried rehmannia root (Radix Rehmanniae), Cyperus tuber (Rhizoma Cyperi), Aucklandia root (Radix Aucklandiae), Prepared rehmannia root (Radix Rehmanniae Praeparata), Chuanxiong rhizome (Rhizoma Ligustici Chuanxiong), White atractylodes rhizome (Rhizoma Atractylodis Mocrocephlae), Liquorice (Radix Glycyrrhizae), Scutellaria root (Radix Scutellariae), Donkey-hide gelatin (Colla corii Asini), White peony root (Radix Paeoniae Alba), Achyranthes and cyathula root (Radix Achyranthis Bidentatae et Radix Cyathulae), Amomum fruit (Fructus Amomi), Poria (Poria)

FUNCTIONS

Nourishing the blood and regulating menstruation.

INDICATIONS

Insuficiency of both blood and Qi, menstrual disorders, abdominal pain during menstruation, soreness and pain of wrist and leg.

DIRECTIONS

To be taken orally, 9g each time, 3 times a day.

PRECAUTION

It should be cautiously used for women in pregnancy.

270 ANKUN ZANYU WAN（安坤赞育丸）

Pill for Multiplying

PRINCIPAL INGREDIENTS

Omission

FUNCTIONS

Reinforing Qi, nourishing blood and regulating menstruation.

INDICATIONS

Insufficiency of blood and deficiency of Qi, menstrua disorder, physical fatigue, metrorrhagia and metrostaxis.

DIRECTIONS

To be taken orally, 9g each time, 1～2 times a day.

It should be cauiously used for women in pregnancy.

271 NU BAO (女宝)

Menstruation-Regulating Capsule

PRINCIPAL INGREDIENTS

Ginseng (Radix Ginseng), Deer foetus (Embryo Cervi), Pilose antler (Cornu Cervi Pantotrichum), Safflowdr (Flos Carthami), Red sage root (Radix Salviae Miltiorrhizae), Moutan bark (Cortex Moutan Radicis), Chuanxiong rhizome (Rhizoma Ligustici Chuanxiong), Donkey-hide gelatin (Colla Corii Asini)

FUNCTIONS

Regulating menstruation and arresting bleeding, warming the womb and arresting leucorrhagia, promoting blood circulation to remove stasis and promoting generation of blood.

INDICATIONS

Irregular menstruation, dysmenorrhea, a-menorrhea, leukorrhagia, sterility due to cold in the womb, abdominal pain after delivery, etc.

DIRECTIONS

To be taken orally, 4 capsules each time, 3 times a day.

PRECAUTION

It is not advisable for pregnant patents. It should be cautiously used for patients with interior heat due to Yin deficiency and in preceded menstrual cycle.

272　ZHI DAI WAN（止带丸）

Leukorrhagia-Relieving Pill

PRINCIPAL INGREDIENTS

Pilose asiabell root (Radix Codonopsis Pilosulae), White atractylodes rhizome (Rhizoma Atractylodis Macrocephalae), Eucommia bark (Cortex Eucommiae), Psoralea fruit (Fructus Psoraleae), Chinese angelica root (Radix Angelicae Sinensis), White peony root (Radix Paeoniae Alba), Chuanxiong rhizome (Rhizoma Ligustici Chuanxiong), Aucklandia root (Radix Aucklandiae), Cyperus tuber (Rhizoma Cyperi), Amomum fruit (Fructus Amomi), Oyster shell (Concha Ostreae), Cockscomb flower (Flos Celosiae Cristatae)

FUNCTIONS

Reinforcing the deficiency of the body to cure leukorrhagia, harmonizing blood to regulate menstruation.

INDICATIONS

Leukorrhagia with white or red discharges, irregular menstruation, abdominal pain and soreness of waist.

DIRECTIONS

To be taken orally, 3~6g each time, 2~3 times a day.

PRECAUTION

It should be avoided to patients with hectic fever due to Yin-deficiency.

273 FUNING SHUAN（妇宁栓）

Suppository for Relieving Woman Diseases

PRINCIPAL INGREDIENTS

Flavescent sophora root (Radix Sophorae Flavescentis), Zedoary (Rhizoma Zedoariae), Catechu (catechu)

FUNCTIONS

Clearing away heat and toxic materials, removing dampness and destroying trichomonad and fungus, removing the necrotic tissue and promoting granulation.

INDICATIONS

Pruritus vulvae, turbid leukorrhea, leukorrhagia with yellow or white discharges, sacralgia and lower abdominal pain.

DIRECTIONS

Clean the pudendum before sleep and push the drug deep into the vagina, once every two days. One course of treatment covers a successive administration of 7 suppositories.

PRECAUTION

Contraindicated for women in pregnancy.

274 FUKE QIANJIN PIAN （妇科千金片）

Prceious Tablet for Gynecology

PRINCIPAL INGREDIENTS

Pilose asiabell root (Radix Coclonopsis Pilosulae), Chinese angelica root (Radix Angelicae Sinensis), Cheroree rose-hip (Fructus Rosae Laevigate), Spatholobus stem (Caulis Spatholobi), Green chiretta (Herba Andrographitis)

FUNCTIONS

Nourishing blood and replenishing Qi, clearing heat and eliminating dampness.

INDICATIONS

Irregular menstruation, abdominal pain, excessive leukorrhea due to inflammation of the genital system.

DIRECTIONS

To be taken orally, 4 tablets each time,

twice a day.

PRECAUTION

It should be cautiously used for women in pregnancy.

275　BAO TAI WAN（保胎丸）

Miscarriage-Preventing Pill

PRINCIPAL INGREDIENTS

Astragalus root (Radix Astragali seu Hedysari), White atractylodes rhizome (Rhizoma Atractylodis Macrocephalae), Liquorice (Radix Glycyrrhizae), Chinese angelica root (Radix Angelicae Sinensis), Prepared rehmannia root (Radix Rehmanniae Praeparata), White peony root (Radix Paeoniae Alba), Chuanxiong rhizome (Rhizoma Ligustici Chuanxiong), Amomum fruit (Fructus Amomi), Macrostem onion (Bulbus Allii Macrostem), Loranthus mulberry Mistletoe (Ramulus Loranthis), Scutellaria root (Radix Scutellariae), Notopterygium root (Rhizoma seu Radix Notopterygii), Schizonepeta (Herba Schizonepetae)

FUNCTIONS

Replenishing Qi and nourishing blood, tonifying kidney and preventing miscarriage.

INDICATIONS

Threatened abortion due to deficiency of both Qi and blood, and deficiency of both spleen and kidnecy.

DIRECTIONS

To be taken orally, 9g each time, twice a day.

PRECAUTION

Avoid cool food.

276 ANTAI WAN (安胎丸)

Anti-Abortion Pill

PRINCIPAL INGREDIENTS

Chinese angelica root (Radix Angelicae Sinensis), White peony root (Radix Paeoniae Alba), White atractylodes rhizome (Rhizoma Atractylodis Macrocephalae), Scutellaria root (Radix Scutellariae), Chuanxiong rhizome (Rhizoma Ligustici Chuanxiong)

FUNCTIONS

Nourishing blood and replenishing Qi, clearing heat and preventing miscarriage.

INDICATIONS

Women in pregnancy, threatened abortion dizziness and vertigo, etc.

DIRECTIONS

To be taken orally, 7～8g each time, twice

a day.

PRECAUTION

It should be cautiously used for patients with spleen-deficiency, loose stool.

277 SHENGHUA TANG (生化汤)

Decoction for Postpartum Troubles

PRINCIPAL INGREDIENTS

Chinese angelica root (Radix Angelicae Sinensis), Chuanxiong Rhizome (Rhizoma Ligustici Chuanxiong), Peach kernel (Semen Persicae), Baked ginger (Rhizoma Zingiberrs), Prepared licorice root (Radix Glycyrrhizae Praeparata)

FUNCTIONS

Promoting blood circulation to remove blood stasis and warming the channels to relieve pain.

INDICATIONS

Retention of lochia after childbirth or scanty amount of discharge of lochia, pain in the lower abdomen with tenderness or with some mass in the sore region.

DIRECTIONS

To be taken orally, 9g each time, 3 times a day.

PRECAUTION

It should be cautiously for women in pregnancy.

278 YIMU PIAN （益母片）
Tablet of Motherwort

PRINCIPAL INGREDIENTS

Motherwort (Herba leonuri), Chinese angelica root (Radix Angelicae Sinensis), Chuanxiong rhizome (Rhizoma Ligustici Chuanxiong), Baked ginger (Rhizoma Zingiberis)

FUNCTIONS

Promoting blood circulation to remove blood stasis and warming the channels to relieve pain.

INDICATIONS

Retention of blood stasis after childbirth, pain of lower abdomen, and abdominal pain during menstruation.

DIRECTIONS

To be taken orally, 3g each time, 3 times a day.

PRECAUTION

Contraindicated for women in pregnancy.

279 CUIRU WAN （催乳丸）
Pill for Promoting Galactorrhea

PRINCIPAL INGREDIENTS

Chinese angelica root (Radix Angelicae Sinensis), Dried rehmannia root (Radix Rehmanniae), Chuanxiong rhizome (Rhizoma Ligustici Chuanxiong), White peony root (Radix Paeoniae Alba), Astrogalus root (Radix Astragali seu Hedysari), Aucklandia root (Radix Aucklandiae), Ricepaper pith (Tetrapanacis), Pangolin scales (Squama Manidae), Vaccaria seed (Semen Vaccariae), Deglued antler powder (Cornu Cervi Degelatiatum)

FUNCTIONS

Replenishing Qi and promoting blood circulation, activating channel to stimulate milk secretion.

INDICATIONS

Deficiency of both Qi and blood after childbirth, galactostasis or hypogalactia.

DIRECTIONS

To be taken orally, 9g each time, twice a day.

280　RUBI XIAO (乳癖消)

Tablet for Nodules of Breast

PRINCIPAL INGREDIENTS

Thallus laminariae (Thallus Eckloniae),

Sar-gassum (Sargassum), Prunella spike
(Spica Prunellae), Moutan bark (Cortex
Moutan Radicis), Red peony root (Radix
Paeoniae Rubra), Scrophularia root (Radix
Scrophulariae), Safflower (Flos
Carthami), Notoginseng (Radix Notogin-
seng), Dandelion herb (Herba Taraxaci),
Spatholobus stem (Caulis Spatholobi),
Deer horn (Cornu Cervi)

FUNCTIONS

Resolving the hard lumps, softening and resolving hard mass. Clearing heat and promoting blood circulation.

INDICATIONS

Nodular mass in the breast, including gy-
necomastia and tuberculosis of breast.

DIRECTIONS

To be taken orally, 1. 6g each time, 3 times
a day.

PRECAUTION

Contraindicated for women in pregnancy.

281 GUIZHI FULING WAN (桂枝茯苓丸)

Pill of Cinnamon Twig and Poria

PRINCIPAL INGREDIENTS

Cinnamon twig (Ramulus Cinnamomi), Poria (Poria), Moutan bark (Cortex Moutan

Radicis), Peach kernel (Semen Persicae),
Red peony root (Radix Paeoniae Rubra)

FUNCTIONS

Removing blood stasis, eliminating mass in
the abdomen.

INDICATIONS

Mass in the abdomen, threatened abortion
during pregnancy, irregular menstruation,
retention of lochia after childbirth, pain in
the abdomen, etc.

DIRECTIONS

To be taken orally, 10g each time, 3 times
a day. If no effect, adds to 20g each time.

PRECAUTION

Contraindicated for pregnant women with
blood stasis.

282 KUSHEN SHUAN (苦参栓)

Suppository of Flavescent

PRINCIPAL INGREDIENTS

Flavescent

FUNCTIONS

Clearing away heat and toxic materials, removing dampness and destroying trichomonad and fungus.

INDICATIONS

Chronic cervicitis, cervical erosion, also ef-

fective in senile vaginitis, colpomycosis, tri-
chomonal vaginitis.

DIRECTIONS

Wash hands and the cunnus before using it,
push it into the depth of the vagina, 1 suppository each time before sleep, once a day,
10 days as one course of treatment.

PRECAUTION

Never to be used in menstrual period.

283 XIAOER NIUHUANG SAN（小儿牛黄散）

Powder of Cow-Bezoar for Children

PRINCIPAL INGREDIENTS

Artificial cow-bezoar (Calculus Bovis Artificiosus)，Musk (Maschus)，Scorpion (Scorpio)，Uncaria sten with hooks （Ramulus Uncariae Cun Uncis），Gastrodia tuber (Rhizoma Gastrodiae)

FUNCTIONS

Clearing away heat，dissolving phlegm，relieving conclusion and calming the endopathic wind.

INDICATIONS

Retention of food and heat in children marked by distention and fullness in stomach and abdomen，constipation due to dryness，tastelessness and convulsion.

DIRECTIONS

To be taken orally，0. 9g each time，twice a day，decreasing relatively in children under one year old.

PRECAUTION

Great care should be taken when exhibiting this drug for the children with loose stool and without heat syndrome.

284 WAN YING DIAG（万应锭）

Troche of Panchrest

PRINCIPAL INGREDIENTS

Artificial cow-bezoar (Calculus Bovis Artificiosus), Musk (Maschus), Borneol (Borneolum), Ox gall (Fel Bovis)

FUNCTIONS

Clearing away heat and toxic materials, calming the endopathic wind and relieving convulsion.

INDICATIONS

Apoplexy, heatstroke, hemiplegia, deviation of the eye and mouth, aphthae, ulcerative gingivitis, swelling and sore in throat. External use in score and furuncle, innominate inflammatory.

DIRECTIONS

To be taken orally, adults: 1. 5g ~ 3g each time; children: the dosage should be reduced accordingly, twice a day. External use, certain dosage should be applied to affected area after mixing with cool boiled - water.

Avoid pungent, hot and greasy foods. Never administered to pregnant women and children with chronic infantile convulsion due to dysfunction of the spleen.

285 XIAOER JIUSOU WAN （小儿久嗽丸）

Pill of Long-Standing Cough for Children

PRINCIPAL INGREDIENTS

Ephedra (Herba Ephedrae), Bitter apricot seed (Semen Armeniacae Amarum), Loquat leaf (Foliu Eriobotryae), Gypsum (Gypsum Fibrosum)

FUNCTIONS

Expelling wind and heat, resolving phlegm and relieving cough.

INDICATIONS

Cough due to heat in the lung with thick and abundant sputum, chronic cough and pertussis.

DIRECTIONS

To be taken orally, under one year old, 1/2 pill each time, twice a day; 1~3 years old, 1 pill each time, twice a day; more than 3 years old, 1 pill every time, three times a day.

PRECAUTION

Fatty, sweat and greasy foods should not be taken.

286   LUSI KA WAN（鹭鸶咯丸）

Pertussis Bolus

PRINCIPAL INGREDIENTS

Ephedra (Herba Ephedrae), Bitter apricot seed (Semen Armeniacae Amarum), Gypsum (Gypsum Fibrosum), Perilla fruit (Fructus Perillae), Trichosanthes peel (Pericarpium Trichosanthis)

FUNCTIONS

Removing and dispersing heat from the lung, resolving phlegm and relieving cough.

INDICATIONS

Infantile pertussis, manifested as persistent cough, dyspnea, hoarseness, hemptysis, chronic edema on face and eyes.

DIRECTIONS

To be taken orally, under one year old, 1/2 pill each time, twice a day; 1～3 years old, 1 pill each time, twice a day; more than 3 years old, 1 pill every time, three times a day.

PRECAUTION

Avoid raw, cold, fatty and sweat food,

contraindicated for pertussis without simul-
taneous occurrence of cold and heat syndromes.

287 NIUHUANG ZHENJING WAN（牛黄镇惊丸）

Cow-Bezoar Bolus for Relieving Convulsion

PRINCIPAL INGREDIENTS

Artificial cow-bezoar (Calculus Bovis Artifi-
ciosus), Arisaema with bile (Arisaema Cum
Bile), Gastrodia tuber (Rhizoma
Gastrodiae), Uncaria stem with hooks (Ra-
mulus Uncariae Cum Uncis), Scorpion
(Scorpio), Batryticated silkworm (Bombyx
Batryticatus)

FUNCTIONS

Removing heat and relieving convulsion,
calming endopathic wind and resolving
phlegm.

INDICATIONS

Infantile convulsion due to acute fever,
short breath, abundant expectoration,
epilepsy induced by terror, trismus, unconsciousness.

DIRECTIONS

To be taken orally, under one year old, 1/2

pill each time, twice a day; 1～3 years old, 1 pill each time, twice a day; 3～7 years old, 1 pill every time, three times a day.

PRECAUTION

Avoid pungent and hot, greasy food.

288 NIUHUANG BAOLONG WAN (牛黄抱龙丸)

Calming Cow-Bezoar Bolus

PRINCIPAL INGREDIENTS

Artipicial cow-bezoar (Calculus Bovis Artificiosus), Scorpion (Scorpio), Batryticated silkworm (Bombyx Batryticatus), Arisaema with bile (Arisaema Cum Bile)

FUNCTIONS

Removing phlegm and calming endopathic wind, clearing away heat and relieving convulsion.

INDICATIONS

Acute infantile convulsion with syndrome of abundant wind-phlegm characterized by abundant expectoration, rapid breathing, coma due to high fever, convulsion, upward staring of the eyes, lockjaws, deep red tongue with little fur, purple superficial venal of index finger.

DIRECTIONS

To be taken orally, 1 pill each time, 2～3 times a day after being infused in warm boiled water or in peppermint decoction. Reducing the dosage accordingly when administered to the children under one year old.

PRECAUTION

Both mothers and children should avoid pungent food. Never administered to the patients of chronic infantile convulsion.

289 ERKE QILI SAN（儿科七厘散）

Infantile Anti-Convulsion Powder

PRINCIPAL INGREDIENTS

Artificial cow-bezoare (Calculus Bovis Artificiosus), Gastrodia Tuber (Rhizoma Gastrodiae), Musk (Moschus), Scorpion (Scorpio), Batryticated silkworm (Bombyx Batryticatus), Uncaria stem with hooks (Ramulus Uncariae Cum Uncis)

FUNCTIONS

Removing heat to arrest convulsion, checking endogenous wind, resolving sputum.

INDICATIONS

Pneumonia, fulminate dysentery and encephalitis B marked as attack of pericardium by heat, coma, restlessness, delirium, recurrent convulsions.

DIRECTIONS

To be taken orally, administered with great care to the children less than six months old. For children of six months to one year old, 1/4 bottle each time, twice a day; 1～3 years old, 1/2 bottle each time, twice a day; 3～7 years old, 1 bottle every time, three times a day. The dosage should be taken after being infused in warm boiled water.

PRECAUTION

The powder should not be taken for a long time, immediate withdraw is indicated once the effect attained.

290 FEIER WAN（肥儿丸）

Fattening Baby Pill

PRINCIPAL INGREDIENTS

Medicated leaven （Massa Fermentata Medicinalis）, Germinated barley （Fructus Hordei Germinatus）, Nutmeg （Semen Myristicae）, Aucklandia root （Radix Aucklandiae）, Quisqualis fruit （Fructus Quisqualis）

FUNCTIONS

Reinforcing the spleen, improving digestion, poisoning and expelling parasites, removing stagnation of food.

INDICATIONS
Infantile indigestion, food retention, malnutrition due to parasitic infestation, etc..

DIRECTIONS
To be taken orally after being infused in warm boiled water during empty stomach, 1～2 pills each time, 1～2 times a day. The dosage should be reduced accordingly when administered to children under three years old.

PRECAUTION
Avoid raw, cold and greasy food.

291 YI NIAN JIN (一捻金)
Indigestion Powder

PRINCIPAL INGREDIENTS
Rhubarb (Radix et Rhizoma Rhei), Parched morning glory Seed (Pharbitis Seed), Scorched areca seed (Semen Arecae), Ginseng (Radix Ginseng)

FUNCTIONS
Improving digestion, removing retention of food, eliminating sputum.

INDICATIONS
Stagnation of water, milk and food in chil-

dren with symptoms of nausea and vomiting, abuand enuresis.

DIRECTIONS

To be taken orally, 0. 6g each time, 1～2 times a day.

PRECAUTION

Never indicated for the patients with diarrhea due to deficiency of spleen and indigestion.

292   BAOCHI SAN（保赤散）

Purging Pill

PRINCIPAL INGREDIENTS

Parched medicated leaven（Massa Fermentata Medicinalis）, Defatted powder of croton seed（Pulvis Crotonis Tiglium）, Arisaema tuber（Rhizoma Arisaematis）

FUNCTIONS

Improving digestion to remove food retention, resolving phlegm and stopping palpitation. ·

INDICATIONS

Infantile cold stagnation, retention of milk and foods, abdominal distention, constipation, palpitation due to fright.

DIRECTIONS

To be taken orally, 6 months to one year

old, 0.09g each time, twice a day; 2～4 years old, 0.18 each time, twice a day; reducing the dosage accordingly when used in children under 6 months. The powder should be taken after infused in sugar boiled water with empty stomach.

PRECAUTION

Avoid cold, raw, greasy foods and difficulty digested food. It should not be used in children with cold, measles and diarrhea. Because there is a drastic herb in this powder, immediate withdraw should be indicated once the effect attained and over-administration is prohibited.

293 BAZHEN GAO（八珍糕）

Cake of Eight Tonics

PRINCIPAL INGREDIENTS

Pilose asiabell root (Radix Codonopsis Pilosulae), Chinese yam (Rhizoma Dioscoreae), Lotus seed (Semen Nelumbinis), Hyacinth bean (Semen Dolichoris), Poria (Poria), Gordon euryale seed (Semen Euryales)

FUNCTIONS

Strengthening spleen and activating the Qi of spleen.

INDICATIONS

Indigestion and infantile malnutrition due to deficiency of the spleen manifested as emaciation, weariness, poor appetite, nausea and vomiting, abdominal distention, loose stool, white and greasy coating, thready and feeble pulse.

DIRECTIONS

To be taken orally, for children 25g each time, 2~3 times a day; reducing the dosage accordingly when used for children under one year old. The drug should be taken with boiled water.

PRECAUTION

Avoid uncooked and greasy foods and hard-digested foods.

294 SAIJIN HUADU SAN (赛金化毒散)

Excellent Toxin-Removing Powder

PRINCIPAL INGREDIENTS

Rhubarb (Radix et Rhizoma Rhei), Coptis root (Rhizoma Coptidis), Artificial ox gall-stone (Calculus Bovis Factitius), Refined realgar (Realgar)

FUNCTIONS

Clearing away heat and toxic materials.

INDICATIONS

Meals, scarlet fever, rubella, chickenpox and aphthae due to accumulation of toxic heat marked by high fever, thirsty, restless with flushed face, thick chickenpox accompanied with cough and asthma or with swollen gum, constipation, dark urine, redden tongue with yellow fur, string and rapid pulse.

DIRECTIONS

To be taken orally with boiled water, 2~3 times a day; for children under one year old, 1/4 packet each time; 1~3 years old, 1/2 packet each time; 3~5 years old, 2/3 packet each time; over 5 years old, 1 packet each time. For external use, applied on the part of ulcer.

PRECAUTION

Indicated with great care to the patients with insufficiency of the spleen and stomach and without fire of excess type.

295 JIANPI FEIER PIAN （健脾肥儿片）

Tablet for Reinforcing the Spleen to Fatten Baby

PRINCIPAL INGREDIENTS

Ginseng （Radix Ginseng）, White atraety-lodes rhizome （ Rhizoma Atractylodis

Macrocephalae）, Poria （Poria）, Chinese
yam （Rhizoma Dioscoreae）, Liquorice
（Radix Glycyrrhizae）

FUNCTIONS

Replenishing Qi and reinforcing the spleen,
regulating the function of the stomach to remove dampness, promoting digestion and
removing stagnated food, clearing away
heat and destroying parasites.

INDICATIONS

Anorexia, vomiting, parasitism and diarrhea due to insufficiency of the spleen and
stomach and retention of foods in middle-
jiao manifested as emaciation with sallow
complexion, indigestion, fullness in the
stomach, eructation and nausea, vomiting
and diarrhea.

DIRECTIONS

To be taken orally with boiled water, 4
tablets each time for children, 3 times a
day; the dosage should be reduced accordingly for baby.

PRECAUTION

The uncooked, cold and greasy foods
should be avoided.

296 WUFU HUADU DAN （五福化毒丹）

Toxin-Removing Bolus

PRINCIPAL INGREDIENTS

Forsythia fruit (Fructus Forsythiae),
Rhiniceros horn (Cornu Rhinocerotis),
Coptis root (Radix Coptidis), Scrophularia
root (Radix Scrophulariae), Dried rehmannia root (Radix Rehmanniae), Red peony
root (Radix Paeoniae Rubra)

FUNCTIONS

Clearing away heat and toxic materials.

INDICATIONS

Ulcerative gingivitis, aphthae and furuncle
due to stagnation of noxious heat with the
symptoms of fever, flushed face, dry
throat, preference of drink more because of
thirsty, red tongue with yellow coating,
rapid pulse.

DIRECTIONS

To be taken orally with boiled water, 1
tablet each time, 2~3 times a day; for children under 3 years old, half dosage each
time; under 1 year, 1/4 dosage each time.

PRECAUTION

Any hot, pungent and stimulating foods
should be avoid for both mothers and children.

297 YINIAO SAN （遗尿散）

Powder for Enuresis

PRINCIPAL INGREDIENTS

Bitter cardamon （Fructus Alpiniae Oxyphyllae）, Seven-lobed yam （Rhizoma Dioscoreae Septemlobae）

FUNCTIONS

Warming up the spleen and kidney, arresting discharge of urine.

INDICATIONS

Infantile enuresis in children over three years old characterized by urinating every night during sleep, 1～2 times or more every night, pale complexion, mental retardation, severely, aversion to cold with cold limbs, lassitude in loin and legs, large amounts of clear urine, pale tongue with thin and white coating, deep, thready and feeble pulse.

DIRECTIONS

To be taken orally with boiled water in empty stomach in the morning or in the evening, 1 packet each time, 2 times a day.

PRECAUTION

Avoid cold foods, keep the body warm.

298 LONGMU ZHUANGGU CHONGJI （龙牡

壮骨冲剂)

Dragon's Bone and Oyster Shell Infusion for Strengthening Bone

PRINCIPAL INGREDIENTS

Drgon's bone (Os Draconis Fossilia Ossis Mastodi), Oyster shell (Concha Ostreae), Tortoise plastron (Plastrum Testudinis), Pilose asiabell root (Radix Codonopsis Pilosulae), Poria (Poria), White atractylodes rhizome (Rhizoma Atractylodis Macrocephalae)

FUNCTIONS

Replenishing Qi and reinforcing the spleen, regulating the function of the stomach, tonifying the kidney and nourishing the vital essence, strengthening the muscles and bones.

INDICATIONS

Infantile malnutrition marked by leanness, pale and sallow complexion, oligotricha, poor appetite; five kinds of retardation in standing, walking, hair-growing, tooth eruption, the faculty of speech, weariness, preference of sleep, restlessness, hyperhidrosis, morbid night crying; five kinds of flaccidity manifested by flaccidity of extremities and mussels, debility of joints, rigid complexion, mental retardation, cold limbs.

DIRECTIONS

To be taken orally with boiled water, 1 packet each time, 2～3 times a day. The dosage should be reduced accordingly when administered to children under one year old.

PRECAUTION

Contraindicated for the patients with fever due to cold.

299 SANHUANG GAO (三黄膏)

Plaster of Three Yellows

PRINCIPAL INGREDIENTS

Scutellaria root (Radix Scutellariae), Coptis root (Rhizoma Coptidis), Phellodendron bark (Cortex Phellodendri), Capejasmine fruit (Fructus Gardeniae)

FUNCTIONS

Removing heat and toxic substances, relieving swelling and astringing carbuncle.

INDICATIONS

Carbuncle, deep-rooted carbuncle, furuncle, ecthyma and scald by hot water or fire due to dampness, heat and fire-toxin marked by redness, swelling, hot and pain in the affected area, effluent of water and pus from the ulcer after rupture, reddened tongue with yellow and greasy coating, rapid and slippery pulse.

DIRECTIONS

External use, wash the affected area clear with normal saline before applying the plaster to it, once a day.

PRECAUTION

Avoid pungent and irritating food during administration.

300 MEIHUA DIANSHE DAN（梅花点舌丹）

Mume Flower Bolus for Boil of the Tongue

PRINCIPAL INGREDIENTS

Toad venom (Venonum Bufonis), Cow-bezoare (Caliulus Bovis), Borneol (Borneolum), Mume flower (Flos Mume), Bear gall (Fel Ursi)

FUNCTIONS

Clearing away heat and toxic materials, promoting blood circulation to relieve swelling, activating tissue regeneration and alleviating pain.

INDICATIONS

Initial stage of carbuncle and furuncle, swelling and pain of gum and throat, aphthae and boil of the tongue, supperactive mastitis and acute mastitis, innominate inflammatory belong to Yang and excess syndrome.

DIRECTIONS

To be taken orally, 3 pills each time, 1～2 times a day, drink a mouthful water then put the pill on the tongue till feeling numbness of mouth, taken it with warm yellow wine or boiled water. For external use, apply it to the affected area after being infused in vinegar.

PRECAUTION

Administered with care to the weak with deficiency syndrome. It is not advisable for the pregnant women. Overdosage is prohibited.

301 QUFU SHENGJI SAN （祛腐生肌散）

Powder for Removing the Necrotic Tissue and Promoting Granulation

PRINCIPAL INGREDIENTS

Red mercuric oxide （Hydrargyri Oxydum Rubrum）, Calomel （Calomeas）, Dragon's bone （Os Craconis Fossilia）, Frankincense （Resina Olibani）, Myrrh （Myrrha）, Lead powder

FUNCTIONS

Removing the necrotic tissue, promoting tissue regeneration.

INDICATIONS

Difficult evacuation of pus after rupture of carbuncle, deep -rooted carbuncle, furuncle, pyogenic infection and ulcerous diseases, or new tissues is head to grow because of the existence of the necrotic tissues, long-standing nonunion of wound.

DIRECTIONS

External use, scatter proper amount of powder on the necrotic tissue of ulcer; or make the powder into medicated thread and insert thread into sinus, once or two times a days.

PRECAUTION

Apply with great care to the parts of eyes and lips because the powder has strong irritation, contraindicated for patients who is allergy to mercury.

302 BADU GAO (拔毒膏)

Semifluid Extract for Drawing out of the Pus

PRINCIPAL INGREDIENTS

Rhubarb (Radix et Rhizoma Rhei), Cape-jasmine fruit (Fructus Cardeniae), Phellodendron bark (Cortex Phellodendri), Fran-kincense (Resina Olibani), Myrrh (Myrrha), Calomel (Calomeas)

FUNCTIONS

Promoting blood circulation to relieve swelling, clearing away heat and toxic materials.

INDICATIONS

Initial stage or stadium suppurationis, furuncle, nail-like boil, carbuncle, phlegm characterized by local redness, swelling and pain, skin fever, or protruding swelling with pus locating in the middle of carbuncle and having wave motion, these symptoms reflect the pathogenesis of domination of heat and toxin, stagnancy of Qi and blood stasis, putrefaction of blood and tissue.

DIRECTIONS

Warm it soft with soft fire, stick it to affected area, once every two days or each day when rupture.

PRECAUTION

Never administrated for the patients with large ulcer or deep pus-pocket, abundant or thin pus, or with red dermatic papular eruption and itching after application.

303 ZIJIN DING (紫金锭)

Zijin Troche

PRINCIPAL INGREDIENTS

Rnoxia root (Radix Knoxiae), Pleione rhizome (Rhizoma Pleionis), Moleplant seed (Semen Euphorbiae Lathyridis), Musk

(Moschus), Realgar (Realgar)

FUNCTIONS

Inducing resuscitation and avoiding turbid pathogenic factor, clearing away toxins to relieve swelling.

INDICATIONS

Carbuncle, swelling, sore, mumps, damp-warm syndrome and infantile convulsion manifested as carbuncle with local redness, swelling, burning and pain, sclerotic swollen parotid gland with pain, summer diarrhea or dysentery, coma, infantile high fever, sputum rumbling in the throat, upper staring of eyes.

DIRECTIONS

For external use, grind a proper amount of the troche with vinegar, then apply it to the affected area, several times a day; for internal use, 1 troche or 2 troches in severe case each time, once or twice a day. Taken it with boiled water after granduncle it or pounding it in a mortar; the dosage should be reduced accordingly when administered for children.

PRECAUTION

It is not advisable for the women in pregnancy; never administered for the aged and the weak.

304   LIANQIAO BAIDU WAN（连翘败毒丸）

Forsythia Fruit Pill for Removing Toxins

PRINCIPAL INGREDIENTS

Forsythia fruit (Fructus Forsythiae), Honeysuckle flower (Flos Lonicerae), Dandelion herb (Herba Taraxaci), Red peony root (Radix Paeoniae Rubra), Cupejaumine fruit (Fructus Gardeniae)

FUNCTIONS

Clearing away heat and toxins, subduing swelling and alleviating pain.

INDICATIONS

Furuncle, nail-like boil and carbuncle, mumps, suppuractive inflammation of cheek, infection with swollen head, herpes with Yang syndrome due to pathogenic wind-heat and fire-toxin.

DIRECTIONS

To be taken orally, 6g each time, twice a day.

PRECAUTION

Contraindicated for the patients with carbuncle accompanied by Yin syndrome or with deficiency of both Qi and blood.

305 XING XIAO WAN (醒消丸)

Pill for Relieving Swelling

PRINCIPAL INGREDIENTS

Realgar (Realgar), Musk (Moschus), Prepared frankincense (Resina Olibani), Prepared murrh (Myrrh)

FUNCTIONS

Promoting blood circulation to remove toxins, subduing swelling to alleviate pain.

INDICATIONS

Prime infection of carbuncle, acute mastitis, nail-like boil, deep-root carbuncle, scrofula due to fire-toxin of viscera and stagnation of Qi and blood stasis with the typical symptoms of redness, swelling, protruding, hardness and pain on the affected area. Without pus and rupture, reddened tongue with yellow coating, rapid and full forceful pulse.

DIRECTIONS

To be taken orally, the dosage should be changed according to the situation of the disease. For adults, 3~9 g each time, 1~2 times a day, with warm wine or boiled water; for children, over 7 years old, half dosage; 3~7 years old, 1/3 dosage.

PRECAUTION

Pungent food and tonic should not be eaten,
contraindicated for women in pregnancy or
patients with carbuncle after rupture or accompanied with pus.

306   ZHENZHU SAN（珍珠散）

Pearl Powder

PRINCIPAL INGREDIENTS

Pearl powder （ Margarita ）, Calcined
dragon's bone (Os Craconis Fossilia), Calcined gypsum （Gypsum Fibrosum）, Calcined abalone shell (Concha Haliotidis),
Musk (Moschus), Borneol (Borneolum)

FUNCTIONS

Removing toxins and the necrotic tissue,
promoting tissue regeneration to cure ulceration.

INDICATIONS

Nail-like boil, sore, carbuncle with slow-
healing ulcer marked by the symptoms as
ulcer with discharge of pus and water, per-
manent existence of pus coating and pus em-
bolus, slow-healing wound due to non regeneration of new tissue.

DIRECTIONS

External use, scatter a proper amount of
powder into the ulcer, overdosage should be

prohibited. Once a day when abundant pus,
once two days when little pus.

PRECAUTION

Contraindicated for the patients of carbuncle
without pus. Never taken orally.

307 KEYIN WAN（克银丸）

Pill for Treating Psoriasis

PRINCIPAL INGREDIENTS

Smilax glabra (Rhizoma Smilacis Glabrae),
Dittany bark (Cortex Dictamni Radicis)

FUNCTIONS

Removing heat and toxic substance, dispelling wind and arresting itching.

INDICATIONS

Psoriasis due to blood-heat and wind-dryness manifested as acute attack, dermatic
erythema and papular, dry scale upon an-
other, continuous itching accompanied by
sore throat, dry mouth, reddened tongue
with rapid pulse.

DIRECTIONS

To be taken orally, for adults, 2 big honey
pills each time or 1 packet of small honey
pill each time, twice a day, the dosage
should be increased properly in severe case,
anymore reduced relatively for children.

PRECAUTION

1. Never administered to peoriasis due to deficiency of blood and wind-dryness marked by faint basis of the affected area, desquamation, long course of disease, pale tongue with threathy pulse.

2. Avoid pungent and tonic food, stimulating or sensitizing food.

3. Protect from fever due to cold, tonsillitis.

4. Never clean the affected area with hot water.

5. Abuse of drug for external use is prohibited.

308 EZHANGFENG YAOSHUI（鹅掌风药水）

Mixture for Tinea Unguium

PRINCIPAL INGREDIENTS

Goldenlarch bark （Cortex Pseudolnricis）, Cnidium fruit （Fructus Cnidis）, Chaulmoogra seed （Semen Chaulmoograe）, Stemona root （Radix Stemonae）, Pepertree （Pericarpium Zanthoxyli）

FUNCTIONS

Destroying parasites, eliminating dampness and arresting itching.

INDICATIONS

Tinea unguium, tinea manuum, tinea pedis and chronic eczema due to pathogenic wind and dampness and invasion of parasites.

DIRECTIONS

External use, apply to the affected area after washing it clean, 3~4 times a day. Remove the loose part of tissue to make the permeation of the mixture easily.

PRECAUTION

It is not advisable for the patients with ulcer never taken orally, avoid contacting with mucous of the eyes, nose and mouth.

309 YANGXUE SHENGFA JIAONANG (养血生发胶囊)

Capsule for Nourishing the Blood and Promoting the Growth of Hair

PRINCIPAL INGREDIENTS

Prepared rehmannia root (Radix Rehmanniae Praeparata), Chinese angelica root (Radix Angelicae Sinensis), Chuanxiong rhizome (Rhizoma Ligustici Chuanxiong), Fleece-flower root (Radix Polygoni Multiflori), Chaenomeles fruit (Fructus Chaenomelis)

FUNCTIONS

Enriching the blood to replenish Yin.

INDICATIONS

Baldness, scalp itching, abundant dandruff, or greasy hair and baldness after sick or delivery due to deficiency of liver and kidney with insufficiency of the blood and wind-dryness.

DIRECTIONS

To be taken orally for 2~3 months, 4 capsules each time, twice a day.

PRECAUTION

Indicated with care for the patients with abdominal distention and loose stool due to insufficiency of the spleen with overabundance of dampness.

310 YICHALING JIAOQI SHUI (一搽灵脚气水）

Excellent Lotion for Tinea Pedis

PRINCIPAL INGREDIENTS

Flacescent sophora root (Radix Sophrae Flavescentis), Sculellaria root (Radix Scutellariae), Isatis leaf (Folium Isatidis), Honeaysuckle flower (Flos Lonicerae), Borneol (Borneolum)

FUNCTIONS

Expelling wind and removing dampness, clearing away toxin and destroying parasites.

INDICATIONS

Various tinea pedis.

DIRECTIONS

External use, for tinea of reratotic style or vesicular style without ulceration, drop the lotion on the affected area with massage; for tinea pedis of macerative style or vesicular style with ulceration, apply the lotion to the affected area, 3~4 times a day.

PRECAUTION

Keep the local clean, never administered for the patients with toxin infection.

311 HUAN YOU (獾油)

Badger Fat

PRINCIPAL INGREDIENTS

Badger fat, Borneol (Borneolum)

FUNCTIONS

Removing heat and toxin, relieving swelling and alleviating pain.

INDICATIONS

1. First or second degree of scald and burn with the symptoms of dermatic erythema, edema, blister, endless pain.
2. Chilblain during winter with local redness, swelling and pain.

3. Burn due to long-term expose to hot environment marked by dermatic reticular erythema and pigmentation, local burning, itching and pain.

4. External hemorrhoids and mixed hemorrhoid with endless pain on anus.

5. Infantile chancre manifested as grayish white scalp dandruff, matt hair easy to be broken or lost, accompanied by itching.

DIRECTIONS

External use, apply directly to the affected area or apply the fat on the ribbon gauze then stick it to the affected area.

312 BAI YAO (白药)

White Drug-Powder

PRINCIPAL INGREDIENTS

(To be omitted)

FUNCTIONS

Arresting bleeding to cure wound, removing blood stasis to regenerate new tissue, clearing away toxic materials to relieve swelling, promoting blood circulation to alleviate pain.

INDICATIONS

1. Traumatic injury: injuries caused by fall

and stumble, contusion, abrasion, sprain and collision usually accompanied by pelidnoma, skin and muscle wound, redness and swelling after fracture; or caused by knives and spears, wound with bleeding, injury of fasciae and bone with severe pain, pale tongue with slippery pulse; or fall down from height with the symptoms of distention of abdomen due to blood stasis inside, unconsciousness, constipation, aunresis, pale tongue with thready pulse.

2. Menorrhagia: Menorrhagia or metrorrhagia and metrostaxis marked by dark purplish with stagnated blood masses, pain in lower abdomen, pain relived after blood masses is expelled.

3. Lochiorrhea: Abundant or persistent lochia after childbirth or artificial abortion characterized by dark red blood with blood masses, pain in lower abdomen with tenderness and guarding, dark-purplish tongue with ecchymoses taut and uneven pulse.

4. Carbuncle and furuncle with swelling, red, burning and pain in the affected area, accompanied by chill and fever,

headache, nausea, reddened tongue
with greasy coating, taut and rapid
pulse or rapid pulse.

5. Epigastralgia marked by pain in the fixed
area with tenderness and guarding, pain
like knife injury or spitting dark-purplish
blood, black stool, or hiccup after drinking water, dark-purplish tongue and
thready and uneven or taut and uneven
pulse.

6. Sore throat with yellow and white puru-
lent secretion, dysphasia chill and fever,
thick greasy fur, slippery and rapid or
taut and rapid pulse.

DIRECTIONS

External or internal use, (1) whatever
symptoms mentioned above, adults: 0.2～
0.3g each time. If the patient is strong or
the injury is severeer, the dosage may be increased properly but the maximum of
dosage should not exceed 0.5g, once every
four hours. In case of no reaction, more
doses should be taken successively. (2) In
case of bleeding wounds and trauma, minor
or severcr, the drug should be taken with
boiled water; in case of swelling, taken
with wine, the proper amount of the drug

can be applied externally to arrest bleeding. (3) For women diseases mentioned above, it should be taken with wine. For excessive menstruation, taken after being infused in boiled water. (4) In case of venenous sores at the primary stage, 0.2~0.3g should be taken internally and a small amount of the powder mixed with wine should be applied to the affected part. For patients with ulcer only oral administration is advised. (5) Children over 2 years old, 0.03g each time; 5 years old, 0.06g each time. (6) One safety pill is contained in each bottle. For severe traumatic injuries, it should be taken with wine (but no more than one safety pill a day). Contraindicated for light injuries and other diseases.

PRECAUTION

Within the first day after taking it, broad beans, fish, sour and cold food should be avoided. Contraindicated for patients in pregnancy.

313　QILI SAN（七厘散）

Anti-Bruise Powder

PRINCIPAL INGREDIENTS

Frankincense（Resina Olibani），Myrrh

(Myrrha), Safflower (Flos Carthami),
Dragon's blood (Resina Draconis), Mush
(Moschus)

FUNCTIONS

Promoting blood circulation to remove
blood stasis, relieving swelling and pain.

INDICATIONS

Traumatic injury, sudden sprain of the lumbar region with chest pain when breathing,
soft tissue injury and fracture, redness,
swelling and pain due to accumulation of
blood stasis, traumatic bleeding. The basic
indication is traumatic bleeding with pelidnoma, inflammatory and stabling pain,
fearing touching, limited acting, or injuries
of soft tissue and fracture with severe pain,
dark-purplish tongue, taut or uneven pulse.

DIRECTIONS

To be taken orally with warm boiled water
or warm rice wine, adults: 0. 2~0. 9g each
time, 1~3 times a day. The dosage for
children should be reduced properly. External use: mix the powder with white spirit
into paste and apply the paste to the affected part; or scatter the dry powder directly
to the wound.

PRECAUTION

Contraindicated for patients in pregnancy, over-dosage should be avoided due to the drastic powder.

314　YUZHEN SAN（玉真散）

Powder with Marvellous Effect

PRINCIPAL INGREDIENTS

Giant typhonium tuber （Rhizoma Typhonii）, Raw arisaema tuber （Rhizoma Arisaematis）, Gastrodia tuber （Rhizoma Gastrodiae）, Ledebouriella root （Radix Ledebouriellae）, Notopterygium root （Rhizoma seu Radix Notopterygii）, Dahurian angelica root （Radix Angelicae Dahuricae）

FUNCTIONS

Expelling wind and removing the phlegm, relieving spasm and pain.

INDICATIONS

Tetanus marked by aversion to cold, fever, bitter-smiling complexion, spasm of facial muscle, lockjaw, even convulsion of extremities, opisthotonus, or traumatic injuries, swelling and pain due to blood stasis.

DIRECTIONS

Internal use, $1 \sim 1.5$g each time, $2 \sim 3$ times a day, with warm rice wine or decoct-

ed with water. External use: mix the powder with rice wine or vinegar into paster
then apply the paster to the affected area, 1
~2 times a day.

PRECAUTION

As a toxicant drug, the dosage for internal
administration should be proper, over-
dosage or long-term administration should
be prohibited. Never administered for wom-
en in pregnancy.

315 HUOXUE ZHITONG SAN（活血止痛散）

Powder for Promoting Blood Circulation
and Alleviating Pain

PRINCIPAL INGREDIENTS

Ground beetle （Eupolyphagaseu Steleopha-
ga）, Notoginseng （Radix Notoginseng）,
Chinese angelica root （Radix Angelicae
Sinensis）, Frankincense （Resina Olibani）

FUNCTIONS

Promoting blood circulation to remove
blood stasis, relieving swelling to alleviate
pain.

INDICATIONS

Swelling and pain due to traumatic injuries
or internal retention of blood manifested as
hematoman, pain, fracture and injury of

soft tissue of lumber, legs, extremities and trunk, or retention of blood due to traumatic injuries inside, or dysmenorrhea, amenorrhea, stance of the blood after childbirth, mass in the abdomen.

DIRECTIONS

To be taken orally with warm rice wine or warm boiled water, twice a day, 1.5~3g each time.

PRECAUTION

It is not advisable for the pregnant women. Administered with great care for the weak.

316   HUISHENG DIYI DAN（回生第一丹）

Excellent Lifesaving Bolus

PRINCIPAL INGREDIENTS

Ground beetle (Eupolyphagaseu Steleophaga), Chinese angelica root (Radix Angelicae Sinensis), Pyrite (Pyrite), Scorpion (Scorpio), Musk (Moschus)

FUNCTIONS

Promoting blood circulation to remove blood stasis, relieving swelling to stop pain, promoting reunion of fractured bones.

INDICATIONS

Soft tissue injury and fracture caused by fall, stumble, contusion and abrasion marked by local hematoma, pain due to blood stasis, ecchymoma, sudden sprain of the lumbar region with chest pain when breathing. Especially for acute traumas.

DIRECTIONS

To be taken orally with warm rice wine or warm boiled water, twice a day, 0. 6g each time.

PRECAUTION

It is not advisable for the pregnant women.

317 JINBUHUANG GAO (金不换膏)

Marvellous Plaster

PRINCIPAL INGREDIENTS

Atractylodes rhizome (Rhizoma Atractylodis), Chaulmoogra seed (Semen Chaulmoograe), Unprepared wild aconite root (Radix Kusnezoff Monkshood), Ledebouriella root (Radix Ledebouriellae), Notoperygium root (Rhizoma seu Radix Notopterygii)

FUNCTIONS

Expelling wind and cold, removing dampness and activating channels and collaterals, promoting blood circulation to stop pain, tonifying the liver and kidney.

INDICATIONS

Arthralgia-syndrome, acute or chronic injury of tissue manifested as pain, swelling, heaviness, soreness and numbness of muscle, soft tissue and joint, worsely difficulty of flexion and extension of joints, swelling and deformation of joints.

DIRECTIONS

External use, clean the affected area with fresh ginger, warm the pastor soft then apply it to the affected area or point, change it every 5～7 days.

PRECAUTION

It should not be applied to the umbilical region of women in pregnancy.

318　KAN GUZHI ZHENGSHENG WAN（抗骨质增生丸）

Anti-Hyperosteogeny Pill

PRINCIPAL INGREDIENTS

Prepared rehmannia root (Radix Rehmanniae Praeparata), Salt-baking cibot rhizome (Rhizoma Cibotii), Desertliving cistanche (Herba Cistachis), Salt-baking glossy privet fruit (Fructus Ligustri Lucidi), Drynaria rhizome (Rhizoma Drynariae)

FUNCTIONS

Tonifying the liver and kidney, strengthening the muscles and bones, nourishing the blood and promoting blood circulation.

INDICATIONS

Hyper plastic spondylitis, cervinal spondy lopathy, calcaneul spur and osteoarthrosis deformans endenmica due to deficiency of the liver and kidney. The indication of administration is soreness and pain of joint, lassitude in the loins and joints, rigidity of the joint, the symptoms worsen when over fatigue, soreness and numbness of extremities or accompanied by dizziness, arrhythmia dim eyesight and tinnitus.

DIRECTIONS

To be taken orally, 1~2 pills each time, 2 ~3 times a day.

PRECAUTION

It is not advisable for the pregnant women, used with care to the patients with exopathogen. Avoid moisture environment and overwork.

319　JIUHUA GAO （九华膏）

Jiuhua Plaster

PRINCIPAL INGREDIENTS

Tale (Talcum), Borax (Borax), Dragon's bone (Os Craconis Fossilia), Sichuan fritil-

lary bulb (Bulbus Fritillariae Cirrhosae),
Borneol (Borneolum)

FUNCTIONS

Removing dampness to cure sores, relieving
swelling and pain.

INDICATIONS

Swelling and pain of internal hemorrhoid,
incarceration of external hemorrhoid and internal hemorrhoid after aperation due to
downward flow of damp-heat marked by
swelling and pain of hemorrhoid, or incarceration of prolapse of hemorrhoid, even
orison and necrosis, yellow or greasy
tongue fur taut and slippery pulse.

DIRECTIONS

Wash the affected area clean with light salt
water then stick the plaster to it, change it
after every defecation.

PRECAUTION

Avoid pungent and stimulating food.

320　ZANG LIAN WAN（脏连丸）

Bolus for Hematochezia

PRINCIPAL INGREDIENTS

Coptis root (Rhizoma Coptidis), Scultllaria
root (Radix Scultellariae), Dried rehmannia
root (Radix Rehmanniae), Sophora fruit

(Fructus Sophorae), Sophora flower (Flos Sophorae)

FUNCTIONS

Clearing away intestine-heat to arrest bleeding, dispelling wind and removing dampness.

INDICATIONS

Hematochezia due to hemorrhoid and anal fissure manifested with hematochezia with bright red blood but without abdominal pain and tenesmus.

DIRECTIONS

To be taken orally with warm boiled water, 1 bolus each time, twice a day. Children over 7 years old, half the dosage; between 3 ~7 years old, 1/3 dosage.

PRECAUTION

Avoid pungent and stimulating food.

321　DIYU HUAIJIAO WAN (地榆槐角丸)

Bolus of Sanguisorba Root and Sophora Fruit

PRINCIPAL INGREDIENTS

Sanguisorba root (Radix Sanguisorbae), Sophora fruit (Fructus Sophorae Sophora flower (Flos Sophorae), Dried rehmannia root (Radix Rehmanniae), Scutellaria root

（Radix Scutellariae）, Rhubarb （Radix et Rhizoma Rhei）

FUNCTIONS

Clearing away intestine-heat to treat hemorrhoid and relaxing the bowels.

INDICATIONS

Hemorrhoid with pain and swelling, anal pain and itching, lematochezia due to hemorrhoid, or stool mixed with bright red blood, accompanied with dry and hot feces, red tongue with thin white or thin yellow coating, taut and rapid pulse.

DIRECTIONS

To be taken orally with warm boiled water, 1 bolus each time, twice a day.

PRECAUTION

Avoid pungent and stimulating food.

322 XIAOZHI SHUAN （消痔栓）

Suppository for Treating Hemorrhoid

PRINCIPAL INGREDIENTS

Calcined drgon's bone （Os Craconis Fos-silia）, Borneol （Borneolum）, Calomel （Calomeas）, Pearl （Margarita）

FUNCTIONS

Astringing to arrest bleeding, relieving swelling and alleviating pain.

INDICATIONS

Internal or external hemorrhoid marked by hematochezia and swelling and pain.

DIRECTIONS

For anal use only, 1 suppository each time.

PRECAUTION

Keep the stool unobstructed during administration, avoid pungent and fried foods.

323 KU ZHI DING (枯痔灵)

Nail-Like Medicine for Making Hemorrhoid Necrosis

PRINCIPAL INGREDIENTS

Arsenolite (Arsenolitum), Realgar (Realgar), Frankincense (Resina Olibani)

FUNCTIONS

Eroding hemorrhoid.

INDICATIONS

Internal hemorrhoid of every stage, internal part of mixed hemorrhoid, anal fistula.

DIRECTIONS

Adopt lateral recumbent position or to expose anus after evacuation of stool or enema, carry out perianal infiltration anesthesia after routine disaffection, then turn over the hemorrhoid outside and sterilize it, fix the hemorrhoid with left index figure and middle finger, hold the end part of the drug with right thumb and index figure and insert the drug as 25~35 degree along parietal long with rotation maneuver into the center of hemorrhoid under mucous from the spot of 0. 3~0. 5cm above dentate line. The depth of insertion of the drug is about 1cm, cut off the superfluous parts to left 1cm long outside and put the lemorrhoid back into the anus. The amount of drugs for administration depend on how many hemorrhoids exist, generally speaking, 4~6 piece for a hemorrhoid, with 0. 3~0. 5cm between every piece, the amount of drug for every insertion should not exceed 20 pieces. Put the drug directly into anal distula when administered to the patients with anal fistrula.

PRECAUTION

Insertion of drug should not be below dentate line; defecation should be prohibited until 24 hours after operation to avoid bleeding due to olisthy of the drug. If herniation of internal hemorrhoid occur after defection, put it back into anus immediately so as to avoid edema and incarceration. Combination with other drugs of hemostat, anti-inflammatory agent and catharsis is necessary. Contraindicated for the patients with acute diseases, severe chronic diseases, acute inflammation of anus and rectum, diarrhea, malignant tumor and those opt to be bleeding.

324 NEIXIAO LUOLI WAN (内消瘰疬丸)

Pill for Treating Scrofula

PRINCIPAL INGREDIENTS

Prunella spike (Spica Prunellae), Sargassum (Sargassum), Trichosanthes root (Radix Trichosanthis), Niter (Nitrum), Clam shell (Concha Meretricis sue Cyclinae), Zhejiang fritillary bulb (Bulbus Fritillariue Cirrhosae)

FUNCTIONS

Removing phlegm to subdue swelling.

INDICATIONS

Scrofula, fleshy goiter, nodules of breast and subcutaneous nodule characterized by abundant or scanty, large or small subcutaneous nodules without any change in color and temperature of skin, usually occur in neck, chin, limbs and back of body.

DIRECTIONS

To be taken orally with warm boiled water,

6~9g each time, twice a day. Children between 7~14 years old, half of the dosage;
between 3~7 years old, 1/3 of the dosage.

PRECAUTION

It is not advisable for the pregnant women.

325 XIAO JIN DAN (小金丹)

Small Golden Pill

PRINCIPAL INGREDIENTS

Prepared wild aconite root (Radix Aconiti
Kusnezoffii), Trogopterus drug (Faeces
Trogopterorum), Sweetgum resin (Resina
Liquidambaris), Earthworm (Lumbricus),
Frankincense (Resina Olibani)

FUNCTIONS

Activating channels and collaterals, promoting blood circulation to remove mass.

INDICATIONS

Scrofula, goiter, subcutaneous nodule,
nodule in breast, tuberculosis of bone and
joint marked by movable dermatic nodule or
cystic without change in color of the skin,
swelling and pain, or non-healing nuclear
with discharge of thin pur, pale tongue with
greasy fur, taunt and thready or thready
and rapid pulse.

DIRECTIONS

To be taken orally with warm boiled water,
0. 6g each time, severe cases: 1. 2g each
time, twice a day. Covered with quilt to induce diaphoresis after taken. For treatment
of tuberculosis of bone and joint with ulcer
or non-healing ulcer: 6g in five days. For
children over 7 years old, 0. 3g each time,
below 7 years old, 0. 15~0. 3g each time.

PRECAUTION

It is not advisable for the pregnant women.

326　YANGHE WAN（阳和丸）

Bolus for Strengthening Yang

PRINCIPAL INGREDIENTS

Prepared rehmannia root (Radix Rehmanni-
ae Praeparata), Antler glue (Colla Cornus
Cervi), Bark of Chinese cassia tree (Corter
Cinnamoni), Ephedra (Herba Ephedrae),
Baked ginger (Rhizoma Zingiberis)

FUNCTIONS

Replenishing Yang and nourishing the
blood, dispelling cold to clear away stagnation, removing phlegm to cultivate the
channels and collaterals.

INDICATIONS

All cellulitis with Yin syndromes tuberculosis of bone and joint, artroncus of knee,

gangrene of finger or tore, osteomylitis of the maxillary bone, pyogenic infection of bone, subcutaneous nodule, nodule in breast and tuberculosis of thoracic wall with syndrome of cold of insufficiency type, especialey Yang insufficiency due to deficiency kidney. The typical symptoms are nodules with unclear flat swelling without root and change in color of the skin, no red and burning sensation in skin, hard to suppurate, rupture and cure, thin watery pus or mixed with flow.

DIRECTIONS

To be taken orally with warm boiled water, 2 pills each time, 2～3 times a day.

PRECAUTION

Contraindicated for patients with carbunele with local red, swelling and pain accompanied with Yang syndrome or excessive syndrome, or with heat symptoms due to Yin insufficiency, or with heat symptoms from cold transformation.

327   QINGLIANG YOU (清凉油)

Plaster of Clearing Heat

PRINCIPAL INGREDIENTS

Peppermint (Herba Menthae), Peooermint

oil (Oleum Menthae), Camphor (Cinnamomum Camphoral Presl), Caphor oil (Oleum Cinnamomum Camphoral), Eucalyptus oil (Oleum)

FUNCTIONS

Expelling heat with drugs in cool poverty, restoring consciousness, alleviating itching and pain.

INDICATIONS

Cold, heatstroke, dizziness due to trailing by bus and train, bite by mosquito and insect, burning and scald, usually manifested as dizziness, headache, vomiting and trousseau.

DIRECTIONS

External use, apply with massage to Taiyang or Yintang point, or affected area.

PRECAUTION

Never apply to the affected area with ulcer, stop administration when red popular or severer itching occur after application, contraindicated in cases who is allergy to this drug.

328 DONGCHUANG LING (冻疮灵)

Marvellous Plaster for Chilblain

PRINCIPAL INGREDIENTS

Crab shell powder, Canphor (Cinnamomum
Camphoral Presl), Vaseline

FUNCTIONS

Subduing swelling to stop itching.

INDICATIONS

Chilblain with pallor at primary stage, then
red swelling, burning pain in the skin or
itching, numbness, etc..

DIRECTIONS

External use, a small amount of the plaster
should be applied to the affected area, several times a day.

V Medicine for the Diseases of Five Sense Organs

五官科类

329 MINGMU DIHUANG WAN （明目地黄丸）

Rehmannia Bolus for Improving Eyesight

PRINCIPAL INGREDIENTS

Prepared rehmannia root (Radix Rehmanniae Praeparata), Dogwood fruit （Fructus Corni ）, Moutan bark （Cortex Mountan Radicis）, Chinese yam （Rhizoma Dioscoreae）, Poria (Poria）, Oriental wafer plantian rhizome （Rhizoma Alismatis）, Wolfberry fruit （Fructus Lycii）, Chrysanthemum flower （Flos Chrysanthemi）, Chinese angelica root （Radix Angelicae Sinensis）, Tribulus fruit （Fructus Tribuli）, Abalone shell (Concha Haliofidis）, White peony root (Radix Paeoniae Alba)

FUNCTIONS

Nourishing the kidney and liver to improve eyesight.

INDICATIONS

Deficiency of the liver-Yin and kidney-Yin，manifested as xenophthalmia，phatophopbia，blurred vision，epiphora induced by wind and night blindness.

DIRECTIONS

To be taken orally, 1 bolus each time, twice a day.

330 SHIHU YEGUANG WAN （石斛夜光丸）

Eyesight-Improving Bolus of Noble Dendrobum

PRINCIPAL INGREDIENTS

Dendrobium （Herba Dendrobil）, Ginseng （Radix Ginseng）, Poria （Poria）, Liquorice （Radix Glycyrrhizae）, Chinese yam （Rhizoma Dioscoreae）, Desertliving cistanche （Herba Cistenchis）, Wolfberry fruit （Fructus Lycii）, Dodder seed （Semen Cuscutae）, Rehmannia root （Radix Rehmanniae）, Prepared rehmannia root （Radix Rehmanniae Praeparata）, Schisandra fruit （Fructus Schisandrae）, Lucid asparagus （Radix Asparagi）, Ophiopogon root （Radix Ophiopogonis）, Bitter apricot kernel （Semen Armeniacae Amarum）, Ledebouridlla root （Radix Ledebouriellae）, Chuanxiong rhizome （Rhizoma Liqustici Chuanxiong）, Bitter orange （Fructus Aurantii）, Coptis rhizome （Rhizoma Coptidis）, Achyranthes root （Radix Achyranthis Bidentatae）,

Chrrysanthemum flower (Flos Chrysan-the-mi), Tribulus fruit (Fructus Tribuli), Gelosia seeds (Semen Cassiae), Buffalo horn (Cornu Bubali), Antelope's horn (Cornu Sargae Tataricae)

FUNCTIONS

Nourishing Yin and supplementing the kidney, removing heat from liver and improving the acuity of vision.

INDICATIONS

Symptoms such as internal oculopathy and poor sight, blurred vision, mydriasis and fear of light caused by deficiency of the liver and kidney as well as hyperactivity of fire due to Yin deficiency.

DIRECTIONS

To be taken orally, 1 bolus each time, twice a day.

331 NIUHUANG YIJIN PIAN (牛黄益金片)

Tablet of Cow-Bezoar for Throat Trouble

PRINCIPAL INGREDIENTS

Phellodendrom bark (Cortex Phellodendri), Artifiilca cow-bezoar (Calculus Bovis Artificiosus)

FUNCTIONS

Clearing away heat and relieving sore

throat, subsiding swelling and arresting pain.

INDICATIONS

Acute and chronic pharyngitis, laryngopharyneal paresthesia.

DIRECTIONS

Holding in the mouth to suck or swallow. Sucking 1~2 tablets each time, 3 times a day. Swallowing 4~6 tablets each time, 3 times a day.

332　ERLONG ZUOCI WAN（耳聋左慈丸）

Nourishing Pill for Deafness

PRINCIPAL INGREDIENTS

Prepared rehmannia root (Radix Rhemanniae Praeparata), Rehmannia root (Radix Rehmanniae), Moutan bark (Cortex Moutan Radicis), Chinese yam (Rhizoma Dioscoreae), Poria (Poria), Oriental water plantain rhizome (Rhizoma Alismatis), Dogwood fruit (Fructus Corni), Chrysanthemum flower (Flos Chrysanthemi), Bupleurum root (Radix Bupleuri), Akebia stem (Caulis Akebiae), Schisandra fruit (Fructus Schisandrae)

FUNCTIONS

Nourishing the liver and kidney, clearing

away fire and subduing the exuberant Yang of the liver.

INDICATIONS

Deficiency of the liver-Yin and kidney-Yin and flaring-up of fire, manifested as dizziness, vertigo, deafness, etc.

DIRECTIONS

To be taken orally, 9g each time, twice a day.

333　QIANBAI BIYAN PIAN（千柏鼻炎片）

Rhinitis Tablet of Climbing Groundsel and Spikemoss

PRINCIPAL INGREDIENTS

Climbing groundsel (Herba Senecionis Scan-dentis), Spikemoss (Herba Selaginellae), Cassia seed (Semen Cassiae), Ephedra (Herba Ephedrae), Notopterygium root (Rhizoma seu Radix Notopterygii), Chuanxiong rhizome (Rhizoma Ligustici Chuanxiong), Dahuiran angelica root (Radix Angelicae Dahuricae)

FUNCTIONS

Relieving inflammation, hypersensitivity and stuffy nose.

INDICATIONS

Stuffy nose, foul nasal discharge, headache, dry throat and mouth caused by a-cute and chronic nose diseases.

DIRECTIONS

To be taken orally, 3~4 tablets each time, 3 times a day.

334 HUO DAN WAN（藿胆丸）

Pill of Cablin Pacholi and Gallbladder

PRINCIPAL INGREDIENTS

Cablin pacholi (Herba Pogostemonis), Pig gall bladder (Gall Bladder)

FUNCTIONS

Clearing away heat and dampness, relieving stuffy nose.

INDICATIONS

Rhinorrhea with terbid discharge usually seen in nasal sinusitis.

DIRECTIONS

To be taken orally, 6g each time, twice a day.

335 KOUQIANG KUIYANG SAN（口腔溃疡散）

Powder for Aphthous Ulcer

PRINCIPAL INGREDIENTS

Nornaol (Borneolum), Natural indigo (Indigo Naturalis), Alum (Alumen)

FUNCTIONS

Clearing away heat and alleviating pain.

INDICATIONS

Aphthouse ulcer.

DIRECTIONS

To be used externally, put proper amount of it in affected part, 3 ～5 times a day.

336 QING DAI SAN (青黛散)

Powder of Natural Indigo

PRINCIPAL INGREDIENTS

Natural indigo (Indigo Naturalis), Coptis root (Rhizoma Coptidis), Peppermint (Herba Menthae), Borneol (Borneolum), Liquorice (Radix Glycyrrhizae), Borax (Borax)

FUNCTIONS

Clearing away heat and toxic materials, subduing swelling and alleviating pain.

INDICATIONS

Swelling and sore throat, ulcerations of the mouth and tongue, swelling and soreness of the gums, etc.

DIRECTIONS

To be used externally, blow proper amount of it in affected part

337 QING GUO WAN （青果丸）

Pill of Chinese White Olive

PRINCIPAL INGREDIENTS

Chinese white olive （Frucuts Canaris）, Honey suckle flower （Flos Lonicerae）, Platycodon root （Radix Platycodi）, Scrophularia root （Radix Scrophulariae）, White peony root （Radix Paeoniae Alba）, Ophiopogon root （Radix Ophiopogonis）, Subprotrate sophora root （Radix Sophorae Subpostratae）

FUNCTIONS

Removing heat and toxic materials, relieving sore throat and promoting secretion.

INDICATIONS

The attack of wind-heat in the body manifested as obstruction in the throat, dryness in the mouth, noarseness or loss of voice, swelling and sore throat.

DIRECTIONS

To be taken orally, 6g each time, 3 times a day.

338 XUANMAI JIEGAN CHONGJI （玄麦桔甘冲剂）

Infusion of Scrophularia, Ophiopogon, Platycodor and Liquorice

PRINCIPAL INGREDIENTS

Scrophularia root (Radix Scrophylariae), Ophiopogon root (Radix Ophiopogonis), Platycodor root (Radix Platycodi), Liquorice (Radix Glycyrrhizae)

FUNCTIONS

Clearing away heat and nourishing Yin, relieving sore throat and alleviating pain.

INDICATIONS

Swelling and sore throat, dryness in the throat and mouth, hoarseness, etc.

DIRECTIONS

To be taken orally, 10g each time, 3 times a day.

339 LIU SHEN WAN (六神丸)

Pill of Six Ingredients with Magical Effect

PRINCIPAL INGREDIENTS

Artificial cow-bezoar (Galculus Bovis), Musk (Moschus), Borneol (Borneolum), Toad venom (Venenum Bufonis), Pearl (Margarita), Realgar (Realgar)

FUNCTIONS

Removing the poisonous substance, relieving inflammation and alleviating pain.

INDICATIONS

Epidemic diphtheria, sore and swelling

throat, scarlatina, unilateral or bilateral tonsillitis, boils, pyogenis infections.

DIRECTIONS

10 pills each time, hold in the mouth until dissolved, twice a day.

PRECAUTION

Not advisable for pregnant women.

340 XIGUA SHUANG (西瓜霜)

Watermelon Frost

PRINCIPAL INGREDIENTS

Watermelon frost, Borneol (Borneolum)

FUNCTIONS

Clearing away heat and toxic materials, subduing swelling and alleviating pain.

INDICATIONS

Sore and swelling throat, swelling and soreness of the gums due to heat and fire in spleen and lung.

DIRECTIONS

To be taken externally, take proper amount of the powder, blow it to the affected area, 2~3 times a day.

341 BING PENG SAN (冰硼散)

Powder of Boras and Borneol

PRINCIPAL INGREDIENTS

Borax （Borax）, Borneol （Borneolum）,
Dried glaubers salt （Natrii Sulfas Exsicca-
fus）

FUNCTIONS

Clearing away fire and toxic materials, subduing swelling and alleviating pain.

INDICATIONS

Swelling and soreness of the gums, ulcerations of the mouth and tongue due to heat
and fire inside the body.

DIRECTIONS

To be taken externally, taken proper
amount of the powder, blow it to the affected area, 2～3 times a day.

342   ZHU HUANG SAN （珠黄散）

Powder of Pearl and Cow-bezoar

PRINCIPAL INGREDIENTS

Artificial Cow-bezoar （Galculus Bovis）,
Pearl （Margarita）

FUNCTIONS

Clearing away heat and toxic materials, removing the necrotic tissue and promoting
granulation.

INDICATIONS

Swelling and sore throat, ulcerations of the
mouth and tongue swelling and soreness of

the gums.

DIRECTIONS

To be taken orally, 0. 6g each time, twice a day. To be taken externally, taken proper amount of the powder, blow it to the affected area, 2~3 times a day.

347 QING YIN WAN（清音丸）

Voice Clearing Pill

PRINCIPAL INGREDIENTS

Sichuan fritillary bulb (Bulbus Fribillariae Clrrhosae), Pueraria root (Radix Puerariae), Snabegourd root (Radix Trrchosanthis), Chebulae fruit (Fructus Chebulae)

FUNCTIONS

Removing evil heat to ease the pain of sore throat, promoting secretion of saliva and quenching thirst.

INDICATIONS

Obstruction in the throat, dryness in the mouth, and hoarseness or loss of voice due to heat in the lung or deficient secretion of saliva.

DIRECTIONS

To be taken orally, 1 ~ 2 pills each time, twice a day.

344 TIE DI WAN (铁笛丸)

Iron Flute Pill

PRINCIPAL INGREDIENTS

Fritillary bub (Bulbus Fritillariae Trrunbergii), Peel of snakegowd (Rericarpium Trichosanthis), Poria (Poria), Liquorice (Radix Glycyrrhizae), Platycodon root (Radix Platycodi), Chebulae fruit (Fructus Chebulae), Scrophularia root (Radix Scrophulariae)

FUNCTIONS

Nourishing the lung and easing the pain of a sore throat, promoting the production of body fluid to relieve thirst.

INDICATIONS

Swelling and sore throat, hoarseness or loss of voice due to heat in the lung of deficiency secretion of saliva.

DIRECTIONS

To be taken orally, 3g each time, 3 times a day.

345 XI LEI SAN (锡类散)

Tin-Like Powder

PRINCIPAL INGREDIENTS

Artificial cow-bezoar (Galculus Bovis),

Pearl (Margarita), Borneol (Borneolum),
Borax (Borax), Natural indigo (Indigo
Waturolis)

FUNCTIONS

Clearing away heat and toxic materials, removing the necrotic tissue.

INDICATIONS

Domination of toxic-heat in the body manifested as swelling and pain in the throat, ulceration in the mouth and on the tongue.

DIRECTIONS

To be taken externally, taken proper
amount of the powder, blow it to the affected area, 2~3 times a day.

PRECAUTION

Avoid pungent food.

346 HOUZHENG WAN (喉症丸)

Pill for Throat Diseases

PRINCIPAL INGREDIENTS

Zsatis root (Radix Zsatidis), Artificial cow-
bezoar (Calculus Bovis Artifiaosus), Borneol (Borneolum), Pig bile (Bilis Porci),
Dried glaubers salt (Natrii Sufas Exsiccatus), Natural indigo (Indigo Naturalis),
Realgar (Realgae), Borax (Borax), Toad
venom (Stceped in mine), (Venenum Bufo-

nis ）, Plant soot （Pulvis Fumi Carbo-
nisafus）

FUNCTIONS

Clearing away heat and toxic materials,
subduing swelling and alleviating pain.

INDICATIONS

Dharyngitis, laryngritis, tonsillitis, etc.

DIRECTIONS

To be taken orally, 5～10 pills each time,
twice a day.

PRECAUTION

Contraindicated for pregnant women.

347 QING YAN PIAN （清咽片）

Tablet for Throat Diseases

PRINCIPAL INGREDIENTS

Scrophalaria root （Radix Scrophulariae）,
Platycodon root （Radix Platycodi）, Liquon-
ice （Radix Glycyrrhizae）, Scutellaria root
（Radix Scutellariae）, Peppermint （Herba
Menthae）, Honeysuckle flower （Flos Loni-
corae）

FUNCTIONS

Clearing away heat and toxic materials, alleviating a sore throat.

INDICATIONS

The attack of wind-heat, manifested as

swelling and sore throat, dry throat, thirsty, etc.

DIRECTIONS

To be taken orally, $2\sim3g$ each time, twice a day.

VI Medicine for Health-Care
保 健 类

348 XIONGSHI WAN（雄狮丸）

Pill for Being "Strong Lion"

PRINCIPAL INGREDIENTS

Ginseng （Radix Ginseng）, Pilose antler （Cornu Cervi Pantotrichun）, Epimedium （Herba Epimedii）, Nux-vomica seed （Semen Strychni）, Toud venom （Venenum Bufonis）

FUNCTIONS

Tonifying kidney and strengthening Yang, replenishing the vital essence and marrow.

INDICATIONS

Impotence, seminal emission and enuresis marked by pale complexion, aversion to cold and coldness in the extremities, coldness and soreness of the loins and knees, spermatorrhoea, pale tongue with fur, deep and thready pulse.

DIRECTIONS

To be taken orally, 3～5 pills each time, 3 times a day.

PRECAUTION

Never administered to the seminal emission
due to hyperactivity of the ministerial fire or
heat-dampness in the lower-jiao.

349   EJIAO（阿胶）

Donkey-Hide Gelatin

PRINCIPAL INGREDIENTS

Donkey-hide gelatin (Colla Corii Asini)

FUNCTIONS

Replenishing blood and arresting bleeding,
nourishing Yin to moisten the lung, preventing abortion.

INDICATIONS

Sallow complexion due to the deficiency of
blood, dizziness, palpitation, vexation, insomnia, dry cough due to Yin insufficiency,
all syndromes of bleeding, vaginal bleeding
during pregnancy.

DIRECTIONS

Melted by heating for oral administration
with water, for adults, 3 ～9g each time, 2
～3 times a day.

PRECAUTION

Administered with great care to those with
the deficiency of the spleen and stomach.

350   BEIQI JING（北芪精）

Oral Liquid of Astragalus Root

PRINCIPAL INGREDIENTS

Astragalus root (Radix Astragali seu Hedysari), Honey (Mel)

FUNCTIONS

Reinforcing the spleen and lung, tonifying Qi to promote the generation of body fluid.

INDICATIONS

Qi deficiency of the spleen and lung, tendency to get wind-cold, deficient epigastrulyia, metrorrhagia and metrostaxis, spontaneous sweating due to superficial deficiency, pale and flabby tongue , feeble pulse.

DIRECTIONS

To be taken orally, 10ml each time, 2 times a day.

PRECAUTION

Avoid raw, cold and greasy food.

351 QIZAO CHONGJI (芪枣冲剂)

Infusion of Astragalus Root and Chinese-Date

PRINCIPAL INGREDIENTS

Astragalus root (Radix Astragali seu Hedysari), Chinese-date (Fructus Ziziphi Jujubae), Poria (Poria), Sputholobus stem extract (Extractum Caulis Spatholobi)

FUNCTIONS

Reinforcing the spleen, tonifying Qi and nourishing blood.

INDICATIONS

Leukopenia, weakness after recovery from disease, hypoimmunity due to deficiency of viscera characterized by dizziness, shortness in breath, weakness, insomnia, dreaminess, aversion to cold, thready or feeble pulse.

DIRECTIONS

To be taken after being infused in boiled water, adults: 15g each time, 3 times a day; children: the dosage should be reduced accordingly.

PRECAUTION

Avoid cold foods.

352 SHIQUAN DABU JIU (十全大补酒)

Tonic Medicated Wine of Ten Ingredients

PRINCIPAL INGREDIENTS

Chinese angelica root (Radix Angelicae Sinensis), Pilose asiabell root (Radix lodonopsis Pilosulae), Bighead atractylodes rhizome (Rhizoma Atractylodis Macrocephalae), White peony root (Radix Paeoniae Alba), Prepare rehmannia root (Radix

Rehmanniae Praeparata)

FUNCTIONS

Reinforcing both Qi and blood, activating the channels and collaterals, nourishing kidney Yang.

INDICATIONS

Consumptive diseases, dizziness, optic atrophy, metrorrhagia and metrostaxis and non-healing of boils. The clinic main symptoms are emuciation, short breath, fatigue, pale or sallow complexion, palpitation and cold limbs.

DIRECTIONS

To be taken orally after warm it before meals, 20~30ml each time, twice a day.

PRECAUTION

Contraindicated for the pregnant women. It's not advisable for the syndromes of Ying-deficiency or heat of excess type.

353 YANGSHEN WAN (洋参丸)

Capsule of Root of American Ginseng

PRINCIPAL INGREDIENTS

Root of American Ginseng (Radix Panacis Quinquefolli)

FUNCTIONS

Reinforcing Qi and nourishing Yin, clearing

away heat of deficiency type, promoting the productionof body fluid to quench thirst.

INDICATIONS

Cough, hemorrhage and consumptive diseases due to deficiency of Qi and Yin marked by irritability, tiredness, thirsty, consumptive disease with seminal emission, cough due to Qi deiciency, sputum mixed with blood, hectic fever, night sweating, sore loins, dizziness, tinnitus, deafness, feverish sensation in the palms and soles, dry throat and mouth, pink tongue, deep and feeble pulse.

DIRECTIONS

To be taken orally, 2 capsules each time, twice a day.

PRECAUTION

Contraindicated for the pregnant women. It's not advisable for the syndromes of heat of excess type.

354 JIANFEI TONGSHENG PIAN (减肥通圣片)

Marvellous Tablet for Reducing Wheight

PRINCIPAL INGREDIENTS

Rhubarb (Radix et Rhizoma Rhei), Talcum powder (Talcum Pulveratum), Exsiccated

sodium sulfate (Natrii Salfas Exsiccatus),
Ephedra (Herba Ephedrae), Capejasmine
fruit (Fructus Cardeniae)

FUNCTIONS

Relieving exterior syndromes by expelling
pathetic wind, purring heat and loosening
the bowels, promoting the flow of Qi to resolve phlegm, removing dampness and
strengthening the spleen.

INDICATIONS

Non-pathogenic obesity.

DIRECTIONS

To be taken orally, 6 tablets each time, 2~
3 times a day, one cause covers 30 days.

355 QINGGONG CHANGCHUN JIAONANG
（清宫长春胶囊）

Qing Court Ever-Young Pill

PRINCIPAL INGREDIENTS

Ginseng (Radix Ginseng), Chinese angelica
root (Radix Angelice Sinensis), White peony root (Radix Paeoniae Alba), Poria (Poria), Oriental water plantarn rhizome (Rhizoma Alismatis), Rehmannia root (Radix
Rehmanniae), Prepared rehmannia root
(Radix Rehmanniae Praparata), Dogwood
fruit (Fructus Corni), Chinese yam (Rhi-

zoma Dioscoreae), Ophiopogon root (Radix Ophiopogonis), Wolfberry fruit (Fructus Lycii), Achyranthes root (Radix Achyranthis Bidentatae), Grassleaved sweetflag rhizome (Rhizoma Acori Graminei), Schisandra fruit (Fructus Schisandrae), Polygala root (Radix Polygalae), Eucommia root (Radix Eucommiae), Dodder seed (Semen Cuscufae), Arborvitae seed (Semen Biotae), Wolfberry bark (Cortex Lycii Radicis), Desertliving cistanche (Herba Cistanchis), Lucid asparragus (Radix Asparagi), Costus root (Radix Aucklandiae)

FUNCTIONS

Replenishing Qi and enriching the blood, tranquilizing the mind, nourishing the Yin and replenishing the essence and marrow, strengthening constitution and resisting senilism.

INDICATIONS

Weakness of the body, insufficiency of vital essence and energy, amnesia, insomnia and impotence.

DIRECTIONS

To be taken orally, 2 ~ 3 capsules each time, 2~3 times a day.

PRECAUTION

It is no advisable for those who have got a cold.

356   QINGGONG SHOUTAO WAN（清宫寿桃丸）

Qing Court Shoutao Pill

PRINCIPAL INGREDIENTS

Walfberry fruit (Fructus Lycii), Rehmannia root (Radix Rehmanniae), Bitter cardamon (Fructus Alpiniae Oxyphyllae), Walnut kernel (Semen Luglandis)

FUNCTIONS

Tonifying the kidney and enriching the primordial energy, strengthening constitution and resisting senilism.

INDICATIONS

Weakness of the body, senile debility, general debility, senilism, etc..

DIRECTIONS

To be taken orally, 10g each time, 2～3 times a day.

Index of Chinese Alphabet
中文汉语拼音索引

（词首数字为正文中排序）

Powder of Indigo and Clam Shell

X

Z

中国中成药（英文版）

主　　编：陈可冀

　　　　※

责任编辑：张碧金
出 版 者：湖南科学技术出版社
印 刷 者：湖南省新华印刷二厂
发 行 者：中国国际图书贸易总公司
　　　　　（中国北京车公庄西路 35 号）
北京邮政信箱第 399 号　邮政编码 100044
（英文版）1997 年（长 36 开）第 1 版第 1 次印刷
ISBN7—5357—2047—1/R·386
03800
14-E-3167P